The
Brain's
Behind It

New knowledge about
the brain and learning

Alistair Smith

'A wise man proportions his belief to the evidence.'

David Hume
An Essay Concerning Human Understanding (1748)

Making sense of making sense!

'Participants will learn how to teach the right-brained learner'
UK training programme for teachers (September 2000)

OR

'You cannot give any one area of the brain any one function – it's just one step up from phrenology!'
Susan Greenfield
Brain Story (2000)
From a talk given at Technology Colleges Trust (March 1999)

'Right now, brain science has little to offer educational practice or policy.'
John T. Bruer
A Bridge Too Far (1997)

OR

'Brain research in time will have a profound effect on how we teach in schools.'
Rita Carter
Mapping the Mind (1999)

'Think of classroom management, not as a social coercion system, but in terms of its biology.'
Robert Sylwester
Brain Expo Conference, San Diego (January 2000)

OR

'I have a richer panoply of things which teach me than simply the connections between my neurons.'
Danah Zohar
Spiritual Intelligence (1999)

'We use only 4 per cent of our brain's potential.'
Mike Hughes
Closing the Learning Gap (1999)

OR

'The myth that we use only 10 per cent of our brain or less derives more from the self-improvement industry than it does from science.'
Stuart Zola
Brain Expo Conference, San Diego (January 2000)

Published by Network Educational Press Ltd
PO Box 635
Stafford
ST16 1BF

© Alistair Smith 2002
Revised edition 2004

ISBN 1 855 39 083 3

Managing Editor: Janice Baiton
Design and Typesetting: Neil Hawkins – Network Educational Press Ltd
Illustrations: Trevor Bounford – www.bounford.com
Cover artwork: Geoff Tompkinson/Science Photo Library

Printed in Great Britain by MPG Books, Bodmin, Cornwall

Contents

PART THREE
The brain's finally behind it

Foreword

The Brain's Behind It began as a project in one millennium and was completed in another. It is an attempt to make sense of what science says about learning from the point of view of someone with little or no scientific training. It endeavours to separate facts, fallacies and fads and to identify scientific findings about learning that are of use to educators, parents and policy makers.

Some of the excitement of writing this book came along with an increasing realization of my own ignorance as I wrote it. I had been caught up in some of the excitement of the brain-based learning movement and made some errors that I am now pleased to correct. This book is a snapshot of what I can find out about the science of the brain and how it relates to learning at this instance. It is now time to conclude. What I thought when I started is not what I think now. If I leave it much later, then my thinking will have slipped from me again.

The scientific activity I describe in this book considers what variables influence our capacity and willingness to learn. Some of the science felt familiar, some I have been persuaded of and some has come as a revelation to me. In the early pages I try to address head on some of the cherished but fallacious ideas that have fuelled what has become known as the 'brain-based learning' movement.

For the purposes of simplicity the use of the term 'learning' in this book is deliberately broad. It includes the idea of 'a permanent and improved change of condition as a result of activation'. Learning is often achieved through 'purposeful and distributed rehearsal'. Learning does not occur without activation at some level but that activation need not be consciously driven. Thus modelling and mimicry are included within my range of learning strategies. So, too, are distributed rehearsal, processing time, focused and diffused thought, demonstrating understanding through varied means and reflection.

When I use terms such as neuroscience in the book, I intend to include all those disciplines whose focus is the study of the brain. This is a caravan of many members. It includes those who work at the cellular level, who work with imaging studies and who deal with clinical dysfunction. It does include neuroscientists, but I try to identify the work of cognitive psychologists separately. I do so for the purpose of distinction between the physical entity of the brain and what we can observe there, and the cognitive functions that its physical changes may lead to. Often brain and mind are confused in the literature of brain-based learning. Both are interconnected! They must be recognized as such, but there is a difference between observable physical changes and conclusions about related behavioural changes.

I have set out to examine factors that influence the development of the human brain and attempt to explain the notion of insult and possible damaging effects on learning capacity. The role of imitation and mimicry and the importance of structured play are described in detail. The importance of multisensory engagement within sensitive periods seems to me as important in acquiring good learning attributes as does appropriate leavenings of emotional security. Stress is good for learning short term but disastrous beyond that. What happens in the brain with practice? Distributed rehearsal is at the heart of any performance improvement, and maybe the place of rote learning ought to be defined. Is all learning of equal value in the brain? Are some experiences dependent and others expectant? If so, then all learning cannot be equal. What happens when we think mathematically? Are the same structures used for looking at pictures as looking at words? Is there a biology to aggression? What about attention? Can there really be a brain that has a deficit in attention? When we age what happens to memory? Would knowing about the degeneration of memory in ageing tell us anything about classroom learning? We are told that men are from Mars and women from Venus and that boys and girls have such different brains we ought to teach them differently. Should we believe these views? Finally, the self-help industry will tell you that your left brain is logical while your right is creative. Is there any truth in this? If not, then why is this myth so pervasive?

I hope to clear up some of these issues and, if not, then certainly to put forward a well-considered view. I cannot say with certainty if educators and brain researchers will ever be able to communicate meaningfully with each other. Perhaps this book will go a little way to furthering the dialogue.

When I had only just started to write this book, a good friend discovered that a tumour the size of a mandarin orange had lodged itself in her brain. She had just arrived on holiday in Vietnam. She was rushed by air taxi to Bangkok and within 24 hours she was operated on. The phenomenal skill of the surgeons saved her life but the prognosis remained gloomy. Some weeks later she was flown home to England and started her recovery. Radiation therapy followed. It was unsuccessful. She had another lengthy and invasive operation. Chemotherapy followed. Again, unsuccessful. This time the operation scooped out what remained of the tumour and some of the secondaries. On recovery, there was some loss of mobility. Movement has since begun to return as health is restored. It would appear there is success. Fifteen months later and she is in the gym with a fixed smile that her friends recognize is uniquely hers.

It is impossible from a distance to begin to get a sense of what 15 months of hope given and removed, of pain and distress, of constantly having to be positive for yourself and for others must be like. It is equally hard to appreciate the skill of the neurosurgeons from around the world in operating again and then again with finer and finer margins and with higher and higher levels of risk. The skill of the surgeons who helped Lorna is built on the accumulation of hundreds of thousands of hours of dedicated research into the workings of the human brain, some, but only some, of which can be described within the pages of this book. I hope that this book whets your appetite to find out more, to support those whose lives are devoted to furthering our knowledge of the brain and its workings, and to try some of the ideas advanced within the book.

The final thing to say is that I am an educationalist first and foremost. My scientific knowledge and training has been acquired in much the same way as the Victorian amateur. If at any time I am guilty of 'phrenological' thinking, then it has arisen as a consequence of enthusiasm rather than hubris. I have tried throughout to triangulate the evidence so it has more than one voice of authority behind it. Where there are omissions I take consolation in knowing that brain science is indeed a developing science but some of the greatest brains are behind it.

Alistair Smith
February 2004

How to use this book

The organization and structure of the book

This book is organized so that it is easy to navigate through. Hopefully it facilitates different ways of reading. It sets out to be of interest to parents, educators and policy makers. It provides an overview of existing scientific research into the workings of the human brain starting with fallacies and fads. This is followed by a body of factual information from which a set of findings and specific recommendations emerge. Throughout the book the fallacies, fads, facts and findings are kept separate.

The introduction poses the question, 'Can brain research tell us anything about learning?' It then attempts to identify a number of especially virulent fallacies and fads.

Parts one and two are more factual and lead in to part three, which contains the findings. Each chapter in parts one and two is broken down into clearly headed sections and is preceded with a summary and a set of questions by section.

Part one is called 'Wired: the development cycle of the learning brain'. It is organized as a crude time line of the brain in development.

Part two is called 'Ready, wire, fire: a model for the learning brain'. It is organized to demonstrate how brain science can be linked to formal learning. The chapters address topical issues.

Part three is called 'The brain's finally behind it'. It contains a set of findings that arise from the book and separate sets of recommendations for parents, educators and policy makers. Part three also includes an extensive list of questions and where to find answers in the book, recommended websites, further reading and a detailed glossary of terms used. A bibliography is organized by section.

Different entry points

The human brain is complex, multifaceted and highly adaptable. So are you. In respect of this, you are provided with a variety of routes through this book. You can, if you choose:

- start at the beginning and work through.

- start with the fallacies and fads. These are listed in the introduction.

- go straight to the findings and recommendations. These are to be found in part three.

- obtain an overview via the illustrations. There are about 60 and they are positioned carefully within each chapter to provide a distillation of the key learning points.

- obtain an overview via the chapter summaries. Each chapter is preceded with a set of summary points by section.

- start with the questions. These are found at the start of each chapter and are collected together in part three.

- start with keywords or topics. These are provided in the index at the back.

- put it on a shelf to gather dust. Promise yourself that you will get round to reading it one day.

Acknowledgements

This book took a long time to research and write and there have been lots of people providing support along the way. Janice Bailon has been very thorough and professional in her editing approach. Jim Houghton has not only given me complete freedom to choose my subject and write about it, but has been able to rise above any pressures in a positive and pleasant way.

Nearer to home, my wife, Ani, made me laugh and my niece, Connie, made me ham and tomato sandwiches. My brother, Ian, a very active man all his life, had a career as an airline pilot ended by a mild heart attack. The sections on the importance of physical stimulation and emotional stability are for his bedside reading. Finally, my dad now resides in my memories, in my heart and in a suitcase full of pictures under the bed, but he is still here helping. In his own way, he provided the motivation to write this book and will be helping with the others to come.

Chapter 1

Introduction

Can brain research tell us anything about learning?

Within the space of two months I attended two events that addressed the question, 'Can brain research tell us anything about learning?' One was in London and the other was in San Diego, USA. They both conveyed fascinating insights into what is fast becoming the 'brain-based learning movement'.

The event in London was a one-day symposium held at the Royal Institution. It was formal, carefully orchestrated and consisted of neuroscientists presenting their position followed by educationalists presenting theirs. Arguments were carefully made, positions were summarized and discussed and the audience were invited to comment. It all took place in the very lecture theatre where Faraday and Davy had, in the eighteenth century, demonstrated their scientific discoveries. It was very British.

The Brain Expo took place at the Paradise Point Resort, San Diego, California. It was very different from the symposium in London. On the first morning 300 delegates warmed up by doing the dance of neural networking. While a presenter demonstrated at the front, we were all encouraged, and found ourselves willingly agreeing, to simulate various neural structures. I was lifted off my seat as I quickly became a myelin sheath. The woman next to me was being DNA when she should have been potentiating at the synapse. As the hysteria rose, I thought back to the wood panelling of the Institution in London and wondered what the suited academics would have made of all this. How readily would they have 'got collectively down' to the neurotransmitter boogie, if at all?

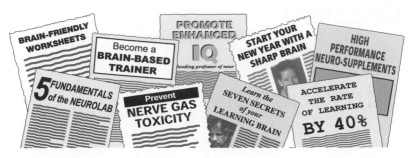

I.I   We are all neurologists – or are we?

Suddenly brain research is sexy. Everyone wants a piece of the action. Courses for teachers with titles like 'Brain-Based Learning' offer their beguiling promise. You can buy teacher packs of 'brain-friendly worksheets'! You can become a licensed 'brain-based trainer'. Training companies with names like Brainsmart, Neurolab and BrainLightning make promises to enhance the performance of students. 'Learn the seven secrets of your learning brain'. These 'seven secrets of your learning brain' look remarkably similar to the 'five fundamentals of the Neurolab', which also bear a striking resemblance to the 'six steps to your lightning brain'. Conference packs are filled with leaflets that implore you to 'start your New Year with a sharp brain'. Another proclaims the benefits of 'high performance neuro-supplements' that not only 'promote enhanced IQ' and 'prevent nerve gas toxicity' but also 'accelerate the rate of learning by 40 per cent'. Yours for only $159.95 for three months supply. What is going on?

What is going on is the coming together of breakthroughs in neuroscience, with powerful non-invasive imaging technologies, powerful computers and the information revolution that is the internet. And, of course, the never-ending educators' quest for a final answer to the question, 'How do we learn?' In the 1970s and 1980s, discoveries in brain science pointed to the possibility of an all-embracing model for learning. A few educators leaped onto this with the adrenaline rush of a lion finding quarry in the Kalahari. Books followed. Careers were realigned. Movements began. Now, for better or worse, the brain-based learning movement is a reality. Or is it simply a fad?

This book attempts to answer this question. Is the enthusiasm for 'brain-based' learning a fad? To what extent does it have a basis in real science? To what extent should those who are interested in the learning of others give it attention? Finally we ask, 'Is it possible, practical and desirable that scientific findings about the brain can enhance learning in the classroom?'

I can save you a lot of reading by telling you now the answers the book provides. They are: 'yes, scientific findings about the brain can be used to enhance learning in the classroom' and 'no, scientific findings about the brain cannot yet be used to enhance learning in the classroom'.

Are we asking the correct questions?

The simple truth is that educators and scientists are asking different questions. The questions they are asking differ in their scope and purpose, their degree of complexity and their level of detail. If you want a rationale for organizing the tables in your classroom, do not go to a neurologist. If you want to know more about a specific piece of laboratory research that may give some clues as to possible causes of a reading disorder, then some of the scientists can help.

Sir Christopher Ball chaired the gathering of teachers and scientists at the Royal Institution, London. The group had come together for a public seminar to examine whether brain science could tell us anything about learning and if so, what. He started the proceedings by posing his own questions.

- ▼ What is the balance between nature and nurture?
- ▼ How important are the early years?
- ▼ Are there special lessons for remedial education and why is remedial education so difficult?
- ▼ Are our links between natural development and artificial education appropriate? Are there differences?
- ▼ What is intelligence?
- ▼ What is emotional intelligence? Can it be developed?
- ▼ How does motivation happen?
- ▼ How far is learning age related?
- ▼ What can be said about different styles of learning?

His questions, posed on behalf of the symposium, are the 'Holy Grail' questions. They are considered and show balance, but they are also general and not susceptible to easy resolution. Finding definitive answers to these questions would transform learning worldwide. Scientists alone cannot provide them.

Educators use the terms 'brain based' and 'brain research' loosely. It is perhaps the educators, more than any other group, who are in search of the 'Holy Grail' answers. Such answers would give a catch-all explanation of how we learn and why. It would provide solace for the teachers who do not know what to do with their low achievers on a wet Friday afternoon. It would stretch and test the academic who wants to test this theory against precedent. Are the answers forthcoming? Yes and no.

In assembling this book, the members of the scientific community whom I have met have expressed not only a passion for learning but also a passion for precision and the specifics. Some of their research into the workings of the human brain reflects the interest of the funding source. Much of the research provides very broad social benefits. All of the research operates at the limits of available technology. It conducts itself within the known cases of, say, brain dysfunction. It cannot generate dysfunction for laboratory purposes. All the research operates within strictly adhered to codes of conduct and ethics. Each and every one of the scientists I talked to or read in preparing this book resisted generalization around their work. This makes it difficult to write!

In writing about learning, Sarah-Jayne Blakemore of University College London, the author of the Early Years Learning paper for the Parliamentary Office of Science and Technology, says

> It is difficult to make direct links between neuroscience and early years education policy.

While at the same time Robert Sylwester, another highly respected commentator on brain science and learning, writes

> Education must change from relying mostly on social and behavioural science to being based more on biology.[1]

John T. Bruer reminds us that the scientific study of the brain and the scientific study of the mind evolved 'separately and independently'. He adds that it is only in the last fifteen years that neuroscience and psychology has seen 'serious collaborative research to study how the biological brain might implement mental processes'. He warns against expecting too much too early,

> Right now, brain science has little to offer educational practice or policy.[2]

This is a bit like suggesting that physics had little to offer computer science. John Stein, Professor of Physiology at Oxford University, disagrees with Bruer, pointing out that advances in the understanding of brain development have already helped pre-school teaching and that cognitive scientists now appreciate that their work depends on an understanding of the brain. In the same year another author writing about the human brain offered a more positive spin,

> Brain research in time will have a profound effect on how we teach in schools.[3]

There is a strong desire within the education community to have science affirm their professional instincts about the complexities of learning. It is an age of rapid breakthrough in brain research. It is also an age where the divisions between disciplines are being questioned and in many cases broken down. Publications emerging from esteemed educators, such as Professor Howard Gardner, draw from different disciplines including neuroscience. Those books that popularize ideas such as emotional intelligence obtain some of their legitimacy by reference to neuroscience. So we have communities looking over the fence at each other. It is an exciting time in the fields of education and in brain research, but it is also a dangerous one.

> ' Politically correct pseudoscience babble.[4] '

Michael Gazzaniga is a highly respected world figure in neuroscience. Here he is writing about the idea that you can 'hot house' your child's language development, and thus intelligence, by an early exposure to the rules of grammar and structured dialogues.[5] It is entirely possible that solid scientific findings are published, translated by an intermediary, popularized, picked up by the media and begin to shape thinking. Before a blink of an eye, every pupil in every school is drinking water, listening to Mozart and rolling their ears between their fingertips. Taking scientific ideas out of context can lead to the creation of damaging pseudoscientific generalizations, which, in turn, can begin to shape policy. It can happen very quickly. I estimate that I have given over 500 separate detailed presentations to diverse audiences in the last five years. I get calls from time to time from the press. The parts that get the attention of the media is the sexy stuff. 'Can you tell us about using classical music in the classroom?' It is never the research that is ringed with caveats and with tight controls. It is never the considered learning model. It is the slightly eccentric but entirely peripheral suggestions sometimes given as an afterthought that catches media interest: visualization of patterns of success as a taught activity, Tai Chi for autistic children, sponsorship for the afternoon sessions from the local fruit and vegetable store.

I have vivid dreams. They are generally favourable. I rarely find myself falling through space, being chased by shadowy figures or drowning in custard. I have in recent months lined up to compete in the Olympic 100 metre hurdles alongside a hippopotamus complete with athletic vest and running shorts. I have also done a lot of surfing, though in reality I've never been on a board. My dreams usually have a narrative, albeit a loose one. They often arrive and leave in snatches with any moral left hanging. Last night it was rats.

The rats were not Orwellian. They were not the product of any phobia, at least none I am aware of. They were laboratory rats and they were pulling covered wagons. The wagons were of the Wild West type and the lab rats were pulling

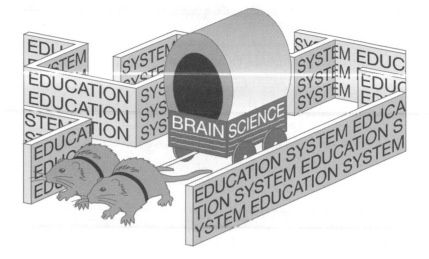

1.2   What influence, if any, will brain science have on our education systems?

them West, pioneer style. What they were doing felt important. There was a lot of authentic Wild West dialogue with words of three letters: 'git', 'yip', 'paw', 'maw'. At one point the rats circled the wagons. The prairie chickens, known for their depravity, were on their way. What happened to the pioneer rats? I never discovered. I awoke early. When I woke, I puzzled as to their fate. Where had that dream come from?

At some point in the last year I had read an article where the author used a metaphor about 'laboratory rats pulling the heavy wagon that is brain science through the maze that is our Western education system', or something similar. It obviously stuck. It is a good metaphor.

Our limited knowledge of human brain function must not be too readily applied to the cognitive potential of children developing in a society with very different demands and expectations than that of their forebears. Brain science alone will not provide the answers but, as ever, educators need to operate in an environment where there is no primer.

Brain science faces problems in answering the questions posed by educators. First there are the broad difficulties:

- Brain science focuses on highly specific questions and educators ask general questions.

- Discovering how a chemical secretes at the synapse does not easily lead to a hypothesis about a learning behaviour and nor is it the scientist's job to make the hypothesis.

- The neuroscience research community is vast and no one individual has an overview.

- Funding influences the research.

- Technology and access to technology influences the research.

- Dysfunction, particularly dysfunction that has a profound community impact, is of more interest than learning.

- Research findings often derive as a consequence of case study, morbidity, invasive surgery, trauma or dysfunction. This is the 'crumbs at the rich man's table scenario'. You get what is left over.

- In the everyday world only laboratory rats live in impoverished environments. You cannot, for the benefit of science, deprive children of stimulation in order to complete research about enriched environments.

- Like any research community, it has its own language and its own means of communicating findings.

Then there are the more specific issues that make it difficult for neuroscientists to answer educators' questions:

 Human brains are different from those of monkeys and rats.

 The brain develops differently in different species.

The brain develops differently in different parts of the brain.

▼ Each brain reflects the environment in which it developed – no two environments are the same (ontogeny reflects phylogeny).

▼ Different modes of learning depend upon different brain systems.

In an age of rapid breakthrough in brain research, the focus needs to remain on the individual child, not on any category of function or dysfunction into which we can fit that child. I am, however, confident that neuroscience offers the promise of a science of individuality rather than that of generality: a science of function rather than dysfunction. Neuroscience offers the possibility of identifying and helping children with conditions that can be clinically defined and recognized. Such conditions can be directly related to learning – dyslexia and dyscalculia – or have a more general effect on a child's willingness or readiness to learn – schizophrenia, depression, autism. As scientists better understand human brain function, the list of conditions that research can identify and help with will expand.

Our understanding of conditions like Attention-Deficit Hyperactivity Disorder, trauma, anxiety and aggression benefit from improved scientific research techniques. This, in turn, can contribute to a shift in perspective away from a ready categorization. The child who is inattentive and can be categorized as 'having' ADHD is the same child who may benefit from more structured variety, more tightly focused and negotiated learning challenges, more physical reprieve and more attention to diet.

The human brain is marvellously plastic while at the same time resilient. It becomes itself through its complexity and responsiveness. Perhaps we can start to respect it by more exacting questions, particularly around fallacies and fads.

Fallacies, fads, facts and findings

It is incumbent on educators to show responsibility in this field, particularly to ask more precise questions of neuroscientists. Follow the instincts of parents in the presence of a doctor. They describe their own child and his quirks of behaviour in elaborate and loving detail. They ask specific questions and give supportive detail. Educators could benefit from a more disciplined and scientific approach to the questions they ask of themselves and of others about their classrooms.

Scientists could benefit from knowing more about the sorts of behaviours that classroom teachers observe on a daily basis. They can help by taking time out to explain the work that they and their colleagues in the field do in a language that is accessible to the lay person.

Educators can help by challenging some of the fallacies that have infiltrated the learning professions from the self-help movement and that have become faddish. For example:

- You only use 10 per cent or less of your brain.
- You have three brains in one.
- Your brain is like a sponge.
- Stress stops you learning.
- You either use it or you lose it.
- Your left brain is logical and your right is creative.
- You have an emotional brain.
- There is a special needs brain.
- Mozart makes you more intelligent.
- Enriched learning environments give your child a better start in life.
- Children can only concentrate for two minutes more than their chronological age.
- The brain cells you get at birth are those you have for life.

- ⇥ There are critical periods within which specific developments must occur.

- ⇥ Genes are destiny.

- ⇥ Your memory is perfect.

- ⇥ Male and female brains are so different we ought to teach boys and girls in different ways.

Sixteen fallacies that fooled us

One: you only use 10 per cent or less of your brain

A UK book for teachers published in 1999 states, 'we use around 2 per cent of our brainpower – this means we waste 98 per cent'. For years, the 10 per cent myth has circulated in the world of self-help psychology. It is a beguiling thought that if there is so much spare capacity, what if we could exploit only 1 or 2 per cent more of it? The truth is that functions such as movement, perception, memory, language and attention are all handled by different areas of the brain. These areas are widely distributed. If you were to lose 98 per cent of your brain, how well would you perform? If 98 per cent is held in reserve, what is it held in reserve for? Should there not be better recovery after trauma? There is no area of the brain that can be damaged without some loss or impairment, however temporary, of function. The brain is highly integrated. For example, imaging studies of sleep show activity in all areas. The problem arose when the self-improvement industry misinterpreted early researchers who said they only knew at most 10 per cent of how the brain functions.

Two: you have three brains in one

Pick a number! This refers to Dr Paul MacLean's triune brain theory. The theory that our brain comprises a primitive or reptilian centre, an emotional and attention centre, and a higher order thinking centre was first discussed in the 1940s and, nowadays, modern researchers would not know anything about it. It has endured because it has a powerful, easily understood metaphorical value and it aligns with Maslow's hierarchy of needs theory. Educators can see the sense in it straight away. The three brains in one theory is not wrong, it is out of date. Science has left it behind.

Three: your brain is like a sponge

This assumes that you take everything in, it is stored somewhere, you have infinite capacity and can draw on that capacity sometime in the future. It is true that your brain probably looks and feels like a sponge, but it never acts like one. Among neuroscientists there is a concept known as neural pruning. As you grow, you reorganize your brain to cope with the demands you place on it. Millions of neural connections that are not put to use get pruned away. If you were to attend to every bit of data that hits your senses, you would not be able to cope with life. To have all your life's accumulated data available is a dysfunction. Selection is part of what the brain does to keep you healthy. Sponges do not select.

Four: stress stops you learning

Partly true! However, it depends on the nature and the duration of the stress, the individual concerned and what is being learned. Short-term, moderate stress is good for learning. Different individuals adapt to anxiety in very different ways. Some 'learning' in stress is so 'successful' that it is impossible to shift thereafter. Post Traumatic Stress Disorder is an example of this. The old thinking used to be that 'downshifting' occurred during stress and higher order thinking was then impossible. Different and more sophisticated models now prevail.

Five: use it or lose it

True – but needs clarification. Active engagement in a task reorganizes the brain, whereas passive stimulation does not do so to anything like the same degree. Learning can and does occur out of conscious awareness but it is not as enduring as that which occurs through active engagement. A further improvement on our understanding of the 'use it or lose it' idea is that the brain is programmed to be experience dependent and experience expectant. In other words, at some stages in our development, some types of experience are more important than others. An adult learning a new language uses different brain structures than a child. The former is dependent and the latter expectant.

Six: your left brain is logical and your right is creative

A seductive idea that has slipped firmly into popular culture. While there is some localization of function, there is no gene, no synaptic connection, no chemical, no area or region, no hemisphere in the human brain that is exclusively responsible for any specific behaviour. Different neural networks within the brain collude with different chemicals to produce responses. Damage the networks or alter the chemicals and you change the responses. Localized damage to one site on either side of the brain can result in loss of function, permanently or temporarily. This does not mean that that site alone was responsible for the function.

Seven: you have an emotional brain

There is a view that we have four basic emotions: anger, sadness, fear and joy. Other emotions are formed from a mix of these. Scientists believe it improbable that one brain structure could run competing emotions. Just as separate but interconnected structures contribute to everyday functions, so it is now thought that different but connected structures contribute to the subtleties of emotional response. Many neuroscientists are sceptical about claims for what is termed 'emotional intelligence' and its links with brain structures.

Eight: there is a special needs brain

There is not a Muslim brain, a white brain, an Inuit brain, a Chelsea Football Club supporter's brain, a shopkeeper's brain or a special needs brain. An individual, particularly a child, should not be labelled by any category of function or dysfunction. It is a wonderful spin-off from brain research that we now know a lot more about very specific cases of dysfunction from which we can begin to generalize. The work at Oxford University on dyslexia and at University College London on autism are good examples. This can help teaching, but it remains a terrifying thought that we should begin to teach a brain rather the child who owns it.

Nine: Mozart makes you more intelligent

No he does not! The Mozart effect is a classic case of the media, with its love of a sexy story and promise of an instant reward, latching on to one research project – which had a limited cohort and a very tightly defined task – and prematurely articulating about it. Not once, but again and again worldwide. Hidden deep behind this there is genuine, quality research. What is of equal interest is how quickly the research can be selected, distorted and re-packaged when there is sufficient public demand. Playing your slumbering infant Mozart piano sonatas is unlikely to do much more than disturb his, and later your, sleep.

Ten: enriched learning environments give your child a better start in life
There is no substantial scientific evidence in support of this. The evidence from laboratory research on rats proves that the absence of a normal environment inhibits learning. It does not prove that *extra* stimulation enhances brain growth, learning and intelligence. Cancel your subscription to *Infant Genius Monthly*, throw away your flash cards and play together the three of you: the baby, you and the cardboard box.

Eleven: children can only concentrate for two minutes more than their chronological age
A maxim that has become accepted as a truth. There is no science behind this. If there were, it would not make such an easy generalization. Buy your 'hyperactive' teenager a Playstation 2 and put it to the test. Human attention varies in its nature. Concentration times are dependent on the individual, the task and the context, not on the chronological age.

Twelve: the brain cells you get at birth are those you have for life
No longer held to be true. Stem cell research and research into neuroplasticity in adults suggest that we can and do grow new brain cells in certain areas of the brain. The hippocampus, an area associated with learning and memory, is one such area.

Thirteen: there are critical periods within which specific developments must occur
This was long held to be true, but has recently been questioned. The correct terminology is now sensitive periods. It is believed that rather than stop abruptly, developmental periods fade away.

Fourteen: genes are destiny
Educators often hear the lament, 'he gets it from his father'. This is usually an apology for a perceived problem or lack of ability. What the boy sees his father do, how the father talks to and around him, and how the father relates to life's challenges, contributes as much to the boy's subsequent behaviour and abilities as his genetic legacy. Genes instruct and guide the body as it develops. Environment acts with genetic inheritance to create a unique brain. Identical twins with the same genes do not have identical brains. The brain alters with use. Adult neuroplasticity is real and remains so right into old age.

Fifteen: your memory is perfect

To quote from a popular text 'there is now increasing evidence that our memories may not only be far better than we ever thought but may in fact be perfect'. Sadly, this is wholly untrue. If you had a perfect memory, your life would be hell. Memory is less about recall than it is about reconstitution. Memories do not reside hidden away in specific sites within the brain. Memory relies on a coming together of a number of variables. Change any of those variables and you change the memory. Memory is by its very nature imperfect! False memory syndrome is real.

Sixteen: male and female brains are so different we ought to teach boys and girls in different ways

Justification for teaching boys and girls in different ways does not come from brain research. Men and women are different, behave differently and have some difference in the organization and structure of their brains. This does not provide a good rationale for education policy. The differences between male and female brains that are reported by many popular texts are exaggerated.

In the remaining sections of this book I try to separate fallacy from fact, locate 'facts' in order to get beyond 'fads' and arrive at some findings. In doing so I recognize that I place my head well and truly above the parapet and am in danger of creating my own set of fallacies and fads. Some shorthand is necessary in a book such as this, but by the time you complete it I hope that Sir Christopher Ball's questions will have had some sort of answer and the fallacies that I believe lead to fads will have received a full and proper correction.

1

PART ONE

Wired: the development cycle of the learning brain

Chapter 2

Pre-wiring:

what happens to the brain in the womb

This chapter contains the following sections:

A quarter of a million cells every minute
How the brain develops from the moment of conception. Why some brain cells are created but will never be used.

Two controlling forces
How learning becomes a 'dance' between genetic inheritance and life experience.

A child inherits its mother's lifestyle
What to do and what not to do during pregnancy. How a child's learning ability can be affected in the womb.

Emotional rescue
When a parent has high levels of anxiety, it can be passed to the child. Hyperactivity in children, especially boys.

Learning and the womb
Is learning possible in the womb? If so, what sort of learning is possible or desirable?

... and will answer the following questions:

- At which point in development does the brain start to become unique?
- To what extent do genes shape destiny?
- What factors in a mother's lifestyle will influence her unborn baby's capacity to learn?
- Does a mother's anxiety in pregnancy pass on to her child?
- Can any learning take place before birth?

Introduction

The Human Genome Project is mapping the 100,000 or so genes that constitute humankind. It is estimated that over half these genes are devoted to producing the brain. Genes are not destiny. Only in a very few cases does a single gene take responsibility for a human disposition. If we are a long way from making a leap from knowledge of brain function to learning behaviours, then we are even further from making the leap from gene to learning behaviour. But it will come![6]

The genes provide broad boundaries for human dispositions, not the dispositions themselves. When a child is born, what has taken place over a period of nine months is a highly complex interactive dance of genes, biochemistry and the environment. A human being is born from a single fertilized egg.

A quarter of a million cells every minute

During every minute of the nine months of pregnancy the brain gains a quarter of a million brain cells. The brain is genetically hard-wired to produce a staggering total of around 100 billion neurons and a trillion glial cells, which provide all the necessary support and protection. This will lead to a multi-trillion network of connections capable of performing 20 million billion calculations per second. At birth, the architecture for supporting vital functions like seeing, hearing, breathing, touching, smelling and tasting is largely in place. The potential for executing those second by second decisions is there.

The brain's development begins with fertilization. DNA from the mother and father combine to form a new cell. Within 24 hours of fertilization, cell division has begun. Three weeks after fertilization, the neural tube forms. The neural tube is the beginning of the central nervous system.

The front end of the tube develops into the brain and the remainder becomes the spinal cord. At around this stage, the cells of the neural tube begin to divide very rapidly. Some of these dividing cells will become neurons (the basic cellular unit in the brain) and some will become glia (a range of cells that support the emerging neural network by providing structure and nourishment).

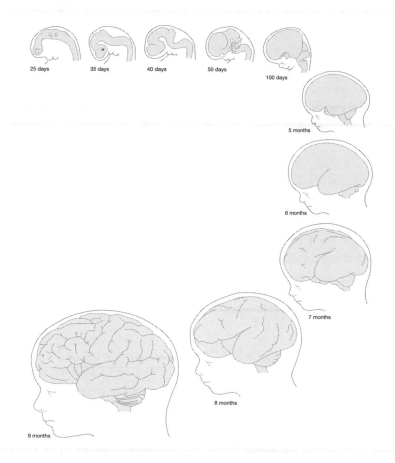

2.1   The development of the human brain from three weeks to nine months showing the forebrain, midbrain and brain stem.

As this process of division continues, cells begin to migrate to positions throughout the developing nervous system. Proper migration of neurons is imperative for the development of a healthy brain. Some learning disorders, including dyslexia, dyspraxia and autism, may be caused in part by migration problems. Over the next few weeks and months, as the cells continue to divide and move, the walls of the neural tube thickens and forms the structures of the cerebral hemispheres, cerebellum, brain stem and spinal cord. Once the migrating neurons reach their destinations, they begin to send out dendrites and axons.

A number of fibres extend from the cell body of the neuron but only one is an axon (a finger-like extension through which the neuron sends out signals). They take signals away from the cell body and can extend for a few metres. The size and quality of the axon determines how fast the impulse travels, which can range from 1 to 150 mph. Repeated use coats the axon in a protective sheath called myelin. This process of myelination makes the transfer of information more efficient so that less neural space is needed.

The neuron sends an electrical signal down its axon to the axon terminals. There is a small gap between the end of the axon and the dendrite of a receiving neuron known as the synapse – from the Greek word for 'union'. Dendrites receive chemical and electrical signals from other neurons. They emerge from many points on the cell body and form relatively short, complex branches. When the axons reach the right dendrites, they form synapses. The synapse is a point where the neurons almost touch and nerve impulses are passed from one neuron to the next via molecules called neurotransmitters. Electrical impulses are changed to chemical at the synapse.

At around the fourth month of pregnancy synapses begin to form. This is when the brain asserts its uniqueness. A single neuron may have thousands of synapses, meaning that within the nervous system there are many trillions of connections between neurons.

As the brain continues its development, it produces more neurons and glial cells than it will need. When the child is born there are twice as many brain cells as there are in the adult brain! Then, in a process that is sometimes described as neural Darwinism, half the cells produced die off. We go from about 200 billion neurons to 100 billion. There are many reasons for this. Some neurons have a function that is temporary and to do with development itself – they do not outstay their usefulness. Other neurons are created for insurance purposes – they hang around to guarantee that all the proper connections are in place. When the proper connections are all ready for that

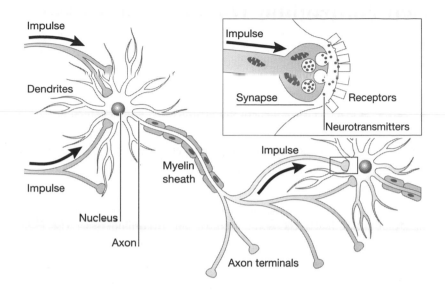

2.2 The major components of the neuron. The cell body or neuron sends an electrical signal down a myelinated axon where it hits a synapse or gap. Here the signal, if strong enough or enduring enough, is converted into a chemical called a neurotransmitter that floats across the gap to a receiving dendrite. If the signal is chemically coded, strong and enduring, it is then passed along to the next neuron.

development stage, any extra neurons are pruned away. When a baby is born all the neurons are in place ready to be stimulated through interaction with the surrounding world.

Early on in utero the brain exhibits torque. It turns in the skull. By 34 weeks the right hemisphere has begun to twist forward and counter-clockwise. The left has twisted back and counter-clockwise. The left hemisphere develops later than the right, particularly in those areas devoted to language. Later in this book the significance of this asymmetry in the brain will be examined.

Two controlling forces

Throughout all of this, two controlling forces exercise their influence. The first is the genes. Inherited from the parents, they direct the development process, telling the cells when to begin their migration and where to travel. The fate of a given cell will depend upon which gene gets activated within its nucleus. For example, when a specific gene called a hox gene is activated in cells of the developing spinal cord, those cells go on to become motor neurons – which send signals to muscle fibres. If a different hox gene is activated, the cells will develop into other cell types.

The other controlling force is the womb itself. According to Dr Lise Eliot, author of *What's Going On in There? How the Brain and Mind Develop in the First Five Years of Life* (1999), 'only in the last few decades has research begun revealing exactly how and when a woman's diet, health, emotional state, and exposure to various environmental agents influence foetal formation.'

Every insult to the mother's health, every threat to her body's homeostasis, every enduring change in her physical well-being is passed on in some way to her unborn child. The crucial time is within the first six weeks. Sadly, in some cases, a woman discovers herself to be pregnant after this period has elapsed and perhaps after smoking or drinking to excess. General lifestyle, health before and during pregnancy, drug and alcohol use, high levels of stress, even exposure to radiation, can all have profound effects on the developing embryo.

Research conducted by Dr Bernie Devlin and reported in *Nature* suggests that the womb environment does contribute to intelligence. The research, conducted in the Department of Psychiatry at Carnegie Mellon University in Pittsburgh, involved a re-analysis of over 200 twin studies. Devlin concluded that the 'impact of genetics on IQ is estimated at 34 per cent.'[7]

Devlin attempted to identify whether there was a 'womb effect' on intelligence. He compared the intelligence scores of twins and sibling pairs and found that twins were much more alike in IQ scores than siblings who are born at different times.

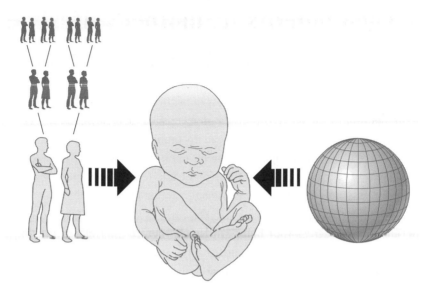

2.3   In a child's development there are two controlling forces. One is the inheritance
from its parents. This includes the genes and the lifestyle factors. The other is the
experience of life itself. This includes factors such as sensory stimulation,
emotional bonding, nourishment and the absence of threat to life and to health.

'There's a womb environment for twins and another for siblings,' he explains,
adding that these are joined by a common home environment to influence
IQ. Factors influencing IQ are subtle and, as he says, 'difficult to pin down'
but there are some obvious factors such as diet, alcohol and drug
consumption.

In the study, Devlin and his colleagues calculated that the womb environment
probably accounts for 20 per cent of the IQ similarity between twins, and
about 5 per cent of the degree of similarity covariance in IQ noted among
brothers and sisters. Some of these studies involved twins separated from
birth who were given IQ tests when they were adults in their 50s, or even in
their 80s.

Devlin and his colleagues say one implication of their study is that
interventions aimed at improving the womb environment 'could lead to a
significant increase in the population's IQ'.

A child inherits its mother's lifestyle

The mother's diet plays a critical role. The food the mother eats supplies all the nutrients available for the developing baby. Unwelcome invaders such as illness, radiation, toxins, drugs or excess of artificial chemicals are likely to be more harmful to the embryo than an impoverished diet. However, shortages of certain nutrients can, and will, lead to problems. Proper closure of the neural tube early in development depends upon the presence of folic acid. A deficiency of folic acid in the mother's diet could lead to improper closure of the tube, resulting in birth defects like spina bifida or anencephaly.

Recent research across four European Union countries correlated low birth weight to subsequent learning difficulties. There was also a correlation between low birth weight and behavioural problems: babies who weighed less than 1.1kg (2.4lb) at birth had a significantly higher incidence of subsequent maladaptive behaviour.

Recent evidence has also associated below normal birth weights with diseases that arise later in life, such as diabetes, breast cancer, obesity and heart disease, all of which were previously thought to be the result of lifestyle and/or genetic predisposition.

Low birth weight can, of course, be caused by a number of factors, many of which are associated with poverty: poor maternal nutrition, ignorance of lifestyle risks, limited access to prenatal care, exposure to certain hormones. In the case of poor nutrition, problems can arise because the foetus will send the available nutrients to the developing brain, at the expense of the other organs.

According to Dr Bradley Peterson, Associate Professor in Child Psychiatry at the Yale Child Study Centre, there are 'dramatic differences' between the brain size of children who were born prematurely and those born at full term. His research involved comparing the brain scans of 25 eight year olds who had been born prematurely with scans from 39 children who were born at full term. The Yale team, whose results were published in the *American Journal of Science*,[8] found that volume in crucial areas of the brain were lower in those born prematurely.

According to Dr Peterson, 'The differences in brain volume on average were dramatic in all regions, with reductions ranging from 11 per cent to 35 per cent. Not all children born prematurely showed these abnormalities, but those born at a younger gestational age were most affected. The magnitudes of the abnormalities in fact were directly proportional to how early the children were born, and they were strongly associated with IQ of the children at age eight years!

'One in ten of all babies born in the UK arrives prematurely! This is why Anne Luther, Director General of the charity Action Research, believes the work is important, 'The Yale study shows that when brains develop prematurely outside of the womb, they are vulnerable to developmental disturbances! Her charity is sponsoring research to 'find out what precisely is responsible for the problems with brain development in these infants!

In both the UK and the USA in recent years there has been an increase in the number of children regarded as having special educational needs. Officially this is often attributed to their needs being better recognized, but some scientists think the improvement in survival rates of premature babies is also a factor.

'Premature birth at less than 1000 grams birth weight (approximately two pounds) is a major cause of developmental disability,' says Dr Laura Ment, Professor of Paediatrics and Neurology at Yale. 'Infants in this birth weight range represent almost 1 per cent of all births in our country, and the survival rate for these infants is well over 80 per cent. But the incidence of handicap is high!

'By age eight years, over 50 per cent are in special education or receiving extensive resource room help. One-fifth have already repeated a grade of school. This study of very low birth weight infants who have been followed since six hours of age provides important insights into the adaptive mechanisms of the developing brain. From these studies, risk factors can be examined and interventions tested!"

The foetus relies entirely on its mother's hormones in the early stages of pregnancy so if a hormonal disorder is present, there can be problems for the child. Researcher Dr Robert Utiger says: 'hypothyroidism in pregnant women can adversely affect their child's subsequent performance on neuropsychological tests'.[10]

Some 17.5 per cent of British women are estimated to suffer from hypothyroidism, which is treatable. It is generally caused by a chronic autoimmune disorder, radioactive iodine therapy, surgery or age-related changes to the thyroid gland. Diet, ethnicity and geography are also thought to play a big part in the disorder. In many developing countries and in communities comprising populations from those countries, iodine deficiency is endemic.

Dr Utiger proposes systematic screening and also that manufacturers should add more iodine to foods such as salt and to all vitamin supplements. Iodine is vital for the production of thyroid hormones. Intake has declined in some Western countries in recent years because people are worried about too much salt in their diet and because manufacturers have reduced the amount of iodine added to bread and animal feed.

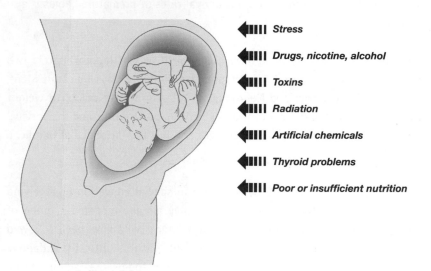

2.4 The womb is designed to be 'womb like'. This means free from illness, radiation, toxins, drugs or an excess of artificial chemicals. Denied key nutrients, a mother's health can suffer and this will in turn lead to difficulties for the unborn child. Proper closure of the neural tube early in development depends upon the presence of folic acid.

Alcohol in the bloodstream during pregnancy can inhibit cell migration. This is a disaster for the unborn child. The brains of alcoholics are smaller than the rest of the population, they are lighter and have less neural density. The brains of babies born to alcoholic mothers show exactly the same symptoms. Foetal Alcohol Syndrome babies have learning and behaviour problems at school, have low IQ scores and are more likely to become alcoholics themselves.

Smoking during pregnancy is one of the biggest threats to the health of the unborn child. The statistics are chilling. Children born to mothers who smoked during pregnancy are 50 per cent more likely to suffer from a cognitive impairment. The risk of spontaneous abortion is 1.7 times higher and the risk of congenital abnormality 2.3 times higher. Babies born to smokers are three times more likely to have a disorder of attention. They are also more likely to have low birth weight. Smaller babies have an increased risk of learning and behavioural problems in later life.

Emotional rescue

Stress for the mother also means stress for the foetus. Stress hormones such as cortisol are released into the bloodstream. Cortisol raises resting heart rate and affects other vital functions as part of the fight or flight response. Exposure in the womb to excessive cortisol could cause problems later in life such as hypertension, quicker stress responses and impaired cognitive abilities. Women who suffer from high levels of anxiety during pregnancy are twice as likely to have a hyperactive child. According to research on 7,000 women by Professor Vivette Glover at Imperial College London, boys were more likely to suffer hyperactivity. The incidence was about 1 in 20 boys, but in women who were highly anxious in pregnancy the figure was nearer 1 in 10.[11]

Professor Glover says her research suggests a chemical element too: 'If the mother is very anxious, her hormone levels change. Some of these hormones, for example cortisol, can cross the placenta and this may affect the development of the baby's brain in the womb.' Another theory is that the mother's anxiety reduces the blood flow to the womb and thus to the baby, cutting the amount of oxygen and nutrients it receives.

Animal studies have shown that exposure to excessive stress hormones before birth may lead to premature ageing of the brain with direct effects on the hippocampus, a brain structure important to learning and memory. As discussed later, the stress response is largely set for life in the womb and in the first few months after birth. Our ability to adapt to, and cope with, unforeseen circumstances is beginning to be laid down before we are born.

Harvard University research led by Dr Mary Carlson found that the emotional bonding between mother and infant changes the infant's brain. Infants who were 'deprived' of what could be deemed normal levels of physical contact and who were put in inadequate nursery provision – characterized by low levels of one-to-one interactions – had abnormal levels of cortisol on weekdays, but not on weekends, when they were home. Such children had the lowest scores on mental and motor testing. Maternal separation causes loss of brain cells in animals such as laboratory rats. If you want to cause stress in a lab rat, deprive it of maternal grooming and suckling. Although the growing brain normally prunes excess synapses and cells, the neurons in the maternally deprived animals die at twice the normal rate.[12]

Stress reducing techniques, such as meditation, may have a positive effect, not just for the mother, but for the developing foetus as well.

Learning and the womb

I watched a television programme about the 'University of the Womb' with fascination and a slight queasiness. Expectant mothers were being encouraged to teach their unborn child 'basic' maths through a combination of light taps and slaps to different parts of their bulging stomachs. As she taps, the mother is being encouraged by an 'expert' to sound out the sums. '*Three* – slap, slap, slap – plus *two* – tap, tap – is *five*' followed by robust and very earnest thumping times five! I could not bring myself to watch to the end. I was too worried about long division.

Dr Lise Eliot, a real expert, points out that the womb is designed to be womb-like! 'There is one feature that best characterizes life in the womb, it is the relative lack of stimulation. The womb, like a sturdy eggshell, is a highly protected environment: dark, warm, confining, and generally quieter than the outside world. This isolation seems to be just the right thing for early brain development' (1999). This conflicts with the view that learning as a result of external stimuli can occur in the womb.

A newly born baby will, within hours, respond to its mother's voice in favour of other voices in the immediate environment. It shows recognition signs. The newborn also responds to its mother's native language in favour of other languages it may be hearing in the immediate environment. It is now believed that all children are born with the capability of learning the sounds of any of the world's languages. This suggests that an unborn foetus may be sensitive to external sounds from within the womb. I met a concert cellist who told me that she played the cello right up to the last week before her daughter was born. At the time she was practising an Elgar piece for a recital she had committed to. She practised the piece daily in the months before her daughter's birth. Fifteen years later her adolescent daughter is still moved every time she hears the music. This had happened from the earliest she can remember.

Despite this, there is no strong evidence that a baby is able to learn in the womb. Some scientists believe prenatal learning, such as exposing the foetus to sound, could prove detrimental, especially if the sounds are invasive, too loud or interrupt the sleep patterns of the developing baby. Sound penetrates the uterus and there is evidence that newborns can recognize sounds heard before birth, but the mechanisms and long-lasting effects of such phenomena remain uncertain.

What do you do to become the perfect parent? I guess what you do is become informed, stay self-aware and relax! Avoid beating yourself up over all the things you do not do and focus on all the things you could do. Lise Eliot (1999) puts it better than I ever could...

> In a perfect world, there's obviously a lot parents could do to improve their children's intellectual prospects. The perfect parent, if she (or he) existed, would devote herself full time to care and teaching of her child. She would begin with, even before conception, by shoring up

her folic acid reserves and purging her body of any chemical remotely suspect. Once pregnant, she would never touch a drop of alcohol, pump her own gasoline, get less than eight hours sleep, or allow herself to be stressed in any way. She would have an ideal, unmedicated, and uncomplicated delivery, and breast-feed from the moment of birth until the child was potty-trained.

She would spend hours every day playing with him – singing, cuddling, talking, massaging, exercising, reading, showing him how all kinds of toys and other fascinating objects work. She'd start him on piano, tennis, dance, French, swimming, art, violin, computer, Spanish, and tumbling lessons at age three, practising herself, to provide a good role model. But this isn't a perfect world. Parenting is hard work. Most of us try the best we can, given the limits on our time, stamina, and resources.

Chapter **3**

Wired to fire:

brain development in the first five years

This chapter contains the following sections:

◈ **Babies learn from the earliest**
How and when a baby begins to make sense of information from the outside world.

◈ **The first learning style: imitation and mimicry**
An area of the brain is devoted to imitation. An explanation of the first learning style and why the mother–child interaction takes place in the way it does.

◈ **The best time to learn any language**
Why talk is so important for a child. Infants store spoken words before they can speak them. Word learning may begin at around eight months.

◈ **Expectancy and dependency**
Some brain growth is programmed. Some is dependent on experience. An explanation of 'sensitive periods'.

◈ **Enriched environments**
Why the idea of enriched environments accelerating learning is flawed. A scientific justification for early emphasis on social interaction, play and exploration.

◈ **Get yourself connected**
An account of how the brain is organized for learning. Why all meaningful learning is about seeking and securing connections.

... and will answer the following questions:

- ⇥ What crucial development takes place at seven months?

- ⇥ Was Piaget too conservative in his estimate of what children can understand in infancy?

- ⇥ What is the best time to learn any language?

- ⇥ Are there 'windows of opportunity' when brain development must occur or be lost forever?

- ⇥ What is the best time for my child to begin formal learning?

- ⇥ Is there an area of the brain that 'does' learning?

Introduction

The brain is the world's most complex, wholly integrated system of interconnected parts. It has phenomenal processing power. Scientists have not got near replicating the brain's unique capacity for managing information. If you are a parent, you have at least one of these complex problem-solving machines lounging in your living room. If you are a teacher, you will have about 30 floating in fluid at an average height of about 1.47m above your classroom floor. Without exaggeration, how those brains experience life in the first five years influences how they will do so forever.

Babies, far from being the empty slates we thought they were, are born with a great deal of understanding. Such 'understandings' can be measured. In part this is because of brain imaging technologies coupled to advanced computers, but it has also come about as a result of what is now considered a more primitive technology: the video camera. Video allows scientists and paediatricians to observe the subtleties of babies' behaviour over extended periods of time and then to replay those recordings, identifying what has been observed and comparing those behaviours with others in the sample. Piaget never had the luxury of a video camera. If he had, would his theories have differed?

Work on how very young babies make sense of the world will, in time, tell us a great deal about learning and about behaviour. Disorders of perception and of attention may arise earlier than was previously thought and may have a real significance in determining our readiness and ability to learn.

Babies learn from the earliest

Babies start to see complex objects in the same way as adults at the age of seven months, according to new research. Using a game like a Pacman called the *Kanizsa Square* and a geodesic sensor, which the baby wears like a swimming hat, scientists discovered that at seven months the brain begins to change the way it perceives objects.

When placed in a particular way, the pieces of the *Kanizsa Square* create the illusion of a square, to the adult brain at least. The scientists wanted to find out when babies start to see the square too. When the babies see the square, the geodesic sensor picks up a burst of brain activity known as a gamma oscillation. The researchers reported in *Science* that they found no sign of the brain signals in six-month-old babies, but did detect it in eight month olds, indicating that the crucial developmental process takes place around the seven-month mark.

Dr Gergely Csibra, leader of a research team from Birkbeck College, said:

> Understanding how an infant brain develops is obviously fascinating and may have implications for the education and care of babies. This new work not only tells us that babies as young as eight months recognize complex objects in the same way an adult does, but also allows us to think of new studies into early infant development. The difference between six- and eight-month-old babies is also intriguing and may show that there is an important development in how the brain organizes information from the outside world at that age.[15]

In the opinion of Professor Alison Gopnik:

> In the last thirty years we have revolutionized what we think about babies and learning.[16]

Scientists, such as Alison Gopnik and those in the Birkbeck team, now believe that powerful learning capacities are evidenced from the earliest. A lab at the University of Washington Obstetrics Unit has been set up so that observations can be made of newborns within minutes of their arrival. In studying babies, scientists look at the pattern of interactions those babies have with the support systems around them that nature has provided – namely adults, parents or carers – and they also look at how information is passed on, interpreted and responded to.

Babies, from the moment they are born, treat humans preferentially. They respond to faces, structures which are made to resemble faces, voices and smells. At birth babies can distinguish between different visual stimuli. Newborn babies get bored and look away when they have been shown the same visual stimulus for some time, and only look again if something new is presented.

Similarly, young babies will listen to their mother's voice longer than a stranger's voice. There is even evidence that babies recognize their mother's voice at birth, from hearing the faint but audible sounds in the womb.[17] Babies recognize their mother's smell. They enjoy 'kangaroo care' – skin to skin. They favour their mother's voice over those of others and they imitate: you stick your tongue out, they stick theirs out; you open your mouth in an exaggerated way, they open theirs. As there are no mirrors in the womb, we can safely assume that the baby has not learned this by seeing itself do it.

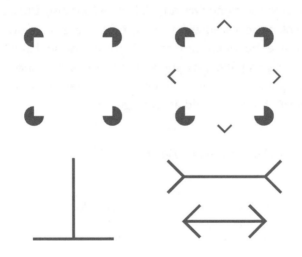

3.1 The Kanisza squares, named after the Italian psychologist Gaetano Kanizsa, are not squares but rather subjective contours. The geometric illusions above show how we view images according to our experience of similar images in real life. The upside-down 'T' looks higher than it is wide. We tend to perceive distances in upward directions differently than we do distances that are horizontal. Upward distances are perceived to be further away than their horizontal equivalents. The topmost images are seen to be bigger. Does it explain why the moon, always a half degree in diameter in the sky, looks bigger when seen close to the horizon?[14]

The baby is somehow linking how it feels on the inside with the emotional responses of others it sees on the outside.[18]

Babies can count! If you show a baby two pieces of card each with a large dot placed in the centre, then slip a blank sheet of card in front and remove it again, the baby stares at the cards. If you do the same thing again but this time add a third dotted piece of card, the baby stares for longer. The baby notices the difference and by its curiosity signals that it has noticed the difference.

The first learning style: imitation and mimicry

Where might a baby learn to imitate? What is the significance of this behaviour for theories of learning? Listen to Professor Alison Gopnik talk on this subject and she points out that there are few, if any, mirrors in the lives of newborns. There are limited opportunities to learn, other than with what already may be there, or through interaction with what is around. What is around mostly tends to be a parent or parents and other adults in the babies' lives.

Within a few days of birth, babies learn to recognize their mother's face – they will look at a picture of their mother's face longer than a picture of a stranger's face.[19] They enjoy watching their mother 'make' faces! Facial expressions are believed to be universal and cross-cultural. The grimaces and face-pulling that comes with the 'parentese' that adults lapse into at the merest sight of a baby could have many functions, and not the least of these functions is an introduction to learning. One of the purposes of imitation is to begin to learn the responses that are necessary to survive in the world of humans. Part of this is to behave like other humans do. Across all primates, mimicry is an important feature of learning in the neonate phase. Through mimicry, neonates explore the functions of their bodies. They begin to distinguish what is internal and what is external. This is part of distinguishing a 'me' from a 'you'. Babies have no way of knowing they are imitating, other than the encouragement they get and a possible kinesthetic sense that it is right. A link is made: you get this nice, reassuring, faintly smelly shape that makes a noise near to you when you do something with your body. It begins to be familiar, you do something you feel inside and the nice, reassuring, smelly thing makes the noise again. It must be right because there it goes again!

There is compelling evidence to show that observing someone making an action activates a component of the brain's motor system to be ready to imitate the action. Areas of the brain that are used to do a task are also used when imagining doing it. Normally an area of the pre-frontal cortex, usually active when you simply watch a task, suppresses the act of imitation. This same area of the brain when damaged causes the patient to mirror and match the behaviour one-to-one. So, I watch you do something such as a physical gesture and the neurons in my brain alert themselves to 'mirror' the gesture you have made but without necessarily completing the gesture.

Work done on non-human primates showed that the pre-motor cortex, an area involved in controlling movement, was activated when the monkey 'observes someone grasping an object, while the monkey makes no movements itself'. The theory of mirror neurons[20] has beguiling promise for educators and points us to the first learning style.[21]

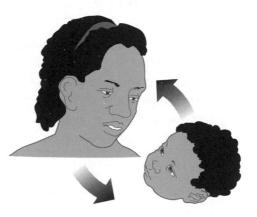

3.2 The interaction between mother and infant shows that you get more of what you reinforce. For some reason 'parentese' includes exaggeration and repetition of sounds and gestures. Is a mother pre-programmed to encourage mimicry in her child?

What role in learning does mimicry or imitation play? Is the role the same in older learners? Authors such as Judith Rich Harris[22] argue a compelling case for the peer group having as much or more influence than the parents in shaping a child's behavioural traits. It is within the peer group that most youngsters learn advanced mimicry and imitation. If you move from one part of the country when your child is very young, the child will quickly abandon mimicking your regional accent in favour of the local one. The theory that any successful behaviour can be broken down into its component parts and 'modelled' is the basis for successful learning techniques such as those of Neuro-Linguistic Programming (NLP).

In humans, scanning techniques show up a similar pattern of neural mirroring as with monkeys. When you or I watch someone make a movement, a part of our brain's motor system is very quickly activated without any corresponding physical movement on our part. Watch two people in rapport in a bar. The more engaged they are with each other the more mimicry occurs. I take a sip of a drink, you quickly follow; I lean back, you do the same; I nod my head, you nod yours. Is this more than showing empathy? Maybe it is part of the learning system for developing understanding of the behavioural patterns of others.[23]

At nine months imitation has already become more sophisticated. In an experiment with a little box with a door that is hinged, the researcher bangs her head in an exaggerated way on the box and the door swings open. This is done several times and the baby is taken away. A week later, when brought back, the baby bangs its head on the box. Bring the baby back a month later and it bangs its head on the box. Some learning has occurred. Some scientists believe that some autistic children lack this fundamental ability to mimic and may be born without it. Alison Gopnik is a philosopher by training and is concerned with the question of mind. At what stage does a baby realize that there are other 'minds'? Piaget believed that such thinking was not possible until well into the school years. Gopnik believes that there is evidence of it from about 18 months.

In experiments done at the University of California at Berkeley by Gopnik, goldfish crackers and broccoli were used to make the breakthrough.[24] The experimenter works with the baby and 'tastes' the goldfish cracker and pulls a face, showing either delight or repulsion. The broccoli is then tried and the 'face' is reversed. The baby is then invited to give the adult some. At 14 months, the baby gives either. At 18 months the baby follows the cue and gives the preferred food. Something happens between 14 and 18 months. The baby develops a sense of a mind other than its own.

We do not yet know whether there are ideal times – what neurologists call sensitive periods – for things like learning maths and reading but we do know that they exist for language.

The best time to learn any language

Japanese native speakers have difficulty in getting their tongue around the sounds 'rah' and 'kah'. They have difficulty recognizing the sounds. However, when they were much younger – and I mean much younger – they could do so successfully. Japanese babies can detect the difference between 'rah' and 'kah' but only before 10–12 months. Because they are not hearing specifically, being babbled at with these sounds, they habituate them out, so that after their first year of life they no longer notice the sound in their environment. Expose children to the sounds of their language through the exaggerated babble of parentese and they become more adept at detecting those sounds. Later these sounds will form the basic building blocks of creating words and, even later, sentences.

Peter Jusczk, a scientist at Johns Hopkins University, discovered why language input is critical before a child even begins to speak or utter any sort of sound.[25] His evidence suggests that infants are using long-term memory to store spoken words before they can speak them. Word learning may begin around eight months, not 12–16 as many parents have thought.

According to Professor John Stein[26] of the University of Oxford nearly two-thirds of the differences in 11-year-old reading ability in the United Kingdom can be explained by poor auditory and visual transient sensitivity. This means that the brain is not yet good enough at tracking subtle changes in sounds, nor in tracking the changing shapes of words represented on a page as the eyes move across that page. Developmental dyslexics are known to be less sensitive to changes in sound frequency and intensity. Illiterate subjects have different patterns of brain activation to literates when asked to do language activities that do not require reading.

We are all born with an equal potential to learn any language. At six months we begin to build the phonemes specific to our native language. Then we get an opportunity to practise manipulating the sounds. With luck we will have a coach who will help us with our manipulations, repeat them, rehearse them and reward our successes with them. We call this coach a parent. A lot of the evidence shows that poor reading skills can be traced in many cases to poor language learning skills and that as many as 30 per cent of children start school with poor language learning skills. Much classroom teaching is language based. Listening to stories helps prepare the brain to be more effective at making its own stories.

The basic unit of language is the phoneme. Learning phonemes starts in the pram or earlier. Children in the bottom 20 per cent in phonological awareness in Year 1 in UK schools are likely to be reading about two and a half years or more below reading age by Year 5. In a project run by Betty Hart and Todd Risley simultaneously in Kansas and in Alaska, four year olds from welfare families were found to have up to 14 million fewer words of cumulative language experience than four year olds from more advantaged blue-and-white and blue collar families.[27] When all socio-economic, class and ethnicity variables were stripped out, what seemed to have made the difference to learning performance was the extent to which the child had encountered language in the first four years of life.

The best three pieces of advice for parents to help their child become a confident reader are:

1 Provide a normal caring home environment with lots of, but not too much, sensory stimulation.

2 Check your child's eyesight, hearing and motor skills.

3 Speak positively, and often, to, with and around your child.

It is in this first four-year period that babies also become explorers and part-time furniture bumpers. They become mobile. This allows them to move towards their desires. They can manipulate their bodies to travel towards objects or people that catch their attention. It is a period of phenomenal neural growth. The provision of safe space in which to explore becomes important. So, too, does the opportunity to practise and to imitate. Babies learn that some things – objects – do not move unless perhaps you propel them, and so are not as much fun to imitate as things that do. Other humans, large and small, are fair game for this. Big humans are instructors in this game, and so are older siblings. Younger siblings, with more instructors, are better at reading minds than older siblings. Mobility necessitates a bigger brain. This is true for birds, it is true for reptiles, it is true for mammals. With increased mobility comes more flexibility in behaviour. Where there is more flexibility, there is need for more brain power to accommodate it.

Expectancy and dependency

Brain development in the early years is both experience–expectant and experience–dependent. This means that certain things are programmed in to happen and other things depend on external stimulation.

An example of experience dependency is given by Professor Nick Rawlins of the University of Oxford.[28] Songbirds' brains change during the breeding season. The acquisition of singing relates to the breeding season. When you do not need to sing, the centres within the brain shrink. The hippocampus is a storage system wherein maps of space are represented in some way. Hippocampal volume in songbirds is seasonal and experience–dependent. Marsh tits store seeds and retrieve them, blue tits do not. Storing birds like marsh tits and magpies have bigger hippocampi than birds like blue tits and jackdaws that do not store. Argentinian cowbirds use lots of nests. The male cowbird visits lots of nests – it gets a larger hippocampus to help it remember where they are. The female sits on the same nest – it loses out. The brain reflects the demands placed upon it.

There are what scientists call 'sensitive periods'. These are windows of opportunity when certain developmental experiences are primed to occur. There are ideal times for the brain to be exposed, through the sensory systems, to sound, to shape and colour, to movement, to tastes, to smells. Missing the window causes problems later in life. These ideal times, the sensitive periods, remain open for a limited period then begin to tail away. The first five years of life contain most, but not all, of the sensitive periods. This is when the adage 'use it or lose it' is most applicable.

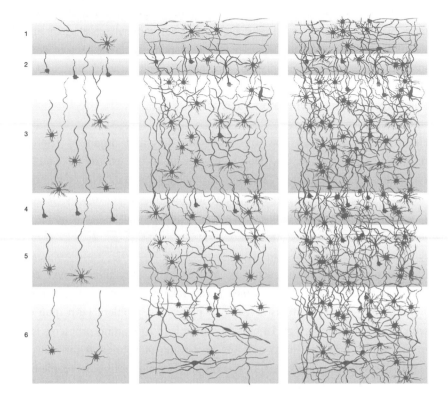

3.3 A cross-section of the cerebral cortex representing the organization of neuronal columns in six layers. Illustrated on the left are typical neurons with cell bodies, axons and dendrites. In the centre, how the cell bodies are distributed. On the right are the neuron fibres and axons. Note how some axons run throughout the layers.

Donald Hebb coined the phrase 'cells that fire together, survive together and wire together'. What he meant was that brain cells are activated by sensory stimulus and by thought, so the more the activation occurs, the more likely it will continue to occur. Prime the connection between brain cells by repeated experience and the cells adapt and become better at responding to the experience. Then the surrounding cells are recruited into the process so that the brain becomes better and better at noticing subtle differences. Columns of neurons assemble themselves together for this purpose. The brain is now wiring in an experience–expectant way in response to the experience. It expects and wants to become good at identifying sounds, seeing shapes and making sense of what is around. As the process continues, what is called 'neural trimming' occurs. If an expected experience does not occur and then does not occur again, eventually the brain goes somewhere else. In other words, the brain cells that were ready to respond to an aspect of sound migrate to another function: 'If I'm not wanted around here, I'll go somewhere where I am!' The study of sensitive periods is important for scientists, parents and educators alike.

For scientists, it shows how the brain develops and organizes itself in response to the world around. No two environments are exactly alike and no two brains are exactly alike. Over time, difference adds to difference and each brain becomes unique. This is what is meant by 'ontogeny reflects phylogeny'.[29] The brain you inherit is a reflection of the use(s) to which it has been put.

For parents, understanding sensitive periods helps in vigilance over their child's health. The best action a parent can take is to monitor the outward signs of the sensory systems at work. A protracted problem with glue ear, which goes undiagnosed at 18 months, could lead to reading problems later in life. All reading has its base in the processing of sounds. A difficulty in separating sounds as a result of a hearing problem will not be overcome by a change in reading scheme.

For teachers, understanding the true nature and purpose of sensitive periods takes them further and further away from the idea of 'hothousing'. In a classic case of mis-using laboratory research with animals, we now have a lobby for hothousing children. The theory goes that because evidence was seen of neural enhancement among laboratory rats put in enriched environments this is a case for enriched environments *per se*.

Enriched environments

At the Salk Institute of Neuroscience in the USA, researchers discovered in 1997 that laboratory rats in an 'enriched environment' grew 15 per cent more neurons in the hippocampus, which, as previously mentioned, is an area of the brain that contributes to visual and spatial memory, than those in the control group. The enriched rats also performed better in maze and intelligence testing. The conclusions included the view that the mechanism for controlling the production and destruction of neural cells is variable, not fixed.[30] This is one study among many that utilizes enriched environments. An enriched environment for a rat in a lab is not one with magazines, sun loungers, a guest-only bar and a whirlpool. An enriched environment contains pipes and tubes to crawl through and around, paper to rummage under, flaps to nudge open and maybe a maze to navigate. In other words, it is a normal environment for a rat! What scientists acknowledge is that 'enrichment studies prove the detriment of extreme deprivation and not the value of enriched environments'. There is no evidence that adding more and more stimulation gives you more and more return in terms of neural capital. But take it away and you very quickly get losses.

For policy makers this is important. A hint of sanity was brought by Sarah-Jayne Blakemore, author of a report to the Parliamentary Office of Science and Technology, London, entitled 'Early Years Learning' (2000). She concluded

> Research suggests that children under the age of four or five may not have fully developed the social and cognitive skills that facilitate learning from formal instruction. Such research has led some to question the value of formal education at an early age and to suggest that a focus on social interaction, play and exploration might be more valuable.

And later,

> There is no convincing evidence that special enriching environments are advantageous to the development of the child.

The answer to the question 'should I hothouse my child?' is no.

Talk to, around and with from the earliest. Use rich language and lots of repetition. Encourage learning behaviours – noticing, naming, describing, speculating, questioning. Encourage physical exploration and robust play. Use lots of imitation and mimicry. Put away your flash cards! Be prepared to be surprised!

The best form of enrichment has to be the security of a positive and supportive relationship with a consistent adult. Harsh words, the abuse of trust, dramatic changes in mood are profoundly harmful to a developing brain.

Abuse in childhood irreparably alters neural development. Work at the McLean Hospital and at Harvard Medical School attempted to find out if childhood abuse might impair the development of the limbic system. The teams were working with patients who, years earlier, had shown up on checklists as having suffered some sort of abuse in childhood.

A significant number of these abused patients showed abnormalities in an area of the cerebellum that released norepinephrine and dopamine, chemicals to do with motivation and reward. Many had a smaller corpus callosum – particularly boys who had been neglected and girls who had suffered sexual abuse. In some there was reduced integration between the right and left hemispheres. Many of these patients showed the symptoms of borderline personality disorder: first placing someone on a pedestal then, as a result of some slight hurt, seeing them as a vindictive enemy, shifting all the while through paranoia to uncontrollable rage. As this happened, brain activity shifted from left to right dominant states with their accompanying different emotional perceptions and memories.

What was happening? The conclusions suggest that early exposure to stress had generated molecular effects that had changed the way in which the developing brain coped with threat. To cope with a world of pervasive threat, the brain needs to be quick to mobilize the survival responses, it needs to prepare for violence without qualm, to be ever vigilant and to be capable of enduring pain and recovering quickly. Thus the brain is in an adapted state – one that will help it survive throughout the reproductive years – but one that is fraught with long-term health risks. Overactivation of stress responses will increase obesity, diabetes, hypertension and psychiatric problems. It will also age the brain more quickly and impair memory function. The brain, always highly adaptable, had been sculpted to exhibit various antisocial behaviours.

In the early years of a child's life the cells in the brain proliferate at a phenomenal rate. Such neural activity will begin to stabilize around puberty. Understanding what goes on is important for parents and educators.

Get yourself connected

Professor Susan Greenfield describes the organization of the human brain like the building of a house.[31] It is the simplest and best analogy I have come across. It works from the smallest unit of function up. Bricks are individually made from basic materials like clay, sand, water and cement. The rooms and floors within the house are built from interconnected walls, comprising bricks, ties and beams. Rooms and floors house obvious functions – living, sleeping, resting and eating spaces – and also less obvious functions – systems for heat, light, water, waste and communications. The house itself has a unique identity and is both functional – 'a machine for living in' – and aesthetic. In many respects, the house is organized in a hierarchy of inter-dependent systems and structures and so is the brain.

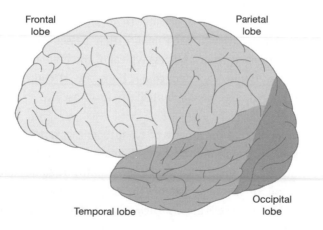

3.4   The major regions of the brain. The cerebral cortex has four lobes each of which contributes to specialized functions. The frontal lobe is involved with planning, disinhibition, decision making and some voluntary movement. The parietal lobe contains sites for speech, touch sensitivity and perception. The occipital lobe contains the primary visual area. The temporal lobe is involved with hearing, speech, smell and aspects of memory.

From bottom up, the brain is organized via the basic unit. This is the brain cell or neuron. The brain cell is shaped by genes and by the presence of chemicals. Brain cells combine together. They do so through electrical and chemical bonds and form circuits. The circuits organize themselves into networks. The networks form large-scale neuronal assemblies. These support specialist brain regions. The specialized regions are supported by whole brain systems, some of which have overlapping functions. The whole is organized into a unique entity. Others look similar – but each is truly unique. This is the equivalent of consciousness. Sometimes the house functions well but occasionally it malfunctions. In such circumstances, we can usually do something about it but every now and again we have to live with the flaws. The brain itself has meaning only when it interacts with others around it. Similarly, with a house. You do not understand it entirely through its occupants, or its bricks, or the type of mortar holding the bricks together, or its wiring. A holistic view is needed. You build your house and then you live in it. Build a good one.

As previously mentioned, a synapse is the physical structure that makes an electrochemical connection between two brain cells. Like many things in life, it is the coming together that makes the difference. The synapse is the mechanism for brain cells connecting together. Synaptic density is the number of synapses per unit volume of brain tissue. Very early on in life, a baby's brain has greater synaptic density than an adult's. Millions of connections are being made with each minute that passes. The process is known as 'synaptogenesis'. Then in a process typical of the brain development of different animals, frequently used connections are strengthened and infrequently used connections are eliminated: use it or lose it.

It is worth remembering that the process of synaptogenesis varies by species, by individual, by brain region and by type of neuron. The brain cells in a baby's head are not all the same, they do not develop to the same timescale, nor do they develop to the same extent. The same is true of 'trimming'. Trimming occurs when brain cells are insufficiently activated and they die off. It is like going to the student ball and not being asked to dance. You hang around for a bit, prepare yourself as best you can, make yourself available to the best – and eventually any – offer and finally go home sheepishly to look for some other distraction. There is not a great deal known about this process of proliferation and pruning of human baby brain cells in the science world because brain tissue can be studied only at autopsy. We do, however, now know more about the development of vision than of any other mental faculty. What has been learned in the last 40 years of research into vision has shown us the general pattern of how the brain wires itself.

The brain devotes more of its space to sight than to all the other senses combined. Researchers have identified at least 32 distinct, tightly organized areas devoted to vision in each hemisphere of the cortex. Each of these areas is highly specialized, servicing a different function of visual recognition. Some areas will be devoted to recognizing vertical lines, some one degree off vertical, some horizontal and so on. Well established evidence exists to show that the eyesight of human babies is enhanced by a very rapid increase in the number of synaptic connections in the first two or three months.[32] It then peaks and plateaux at eight to ten months before declining and then stabilizes at around age ten years. The brain cells adapted to eyesight then stay at this level thereafter. If you are a parent of a newborn, keep in close contact with your local clinic and monitor your child's eyesight, particularly in the first ten months.

The way the brain becomes wired shapes our personality and plays no small part in determining our future. For the Salk Institute, this means recognizing the importance of shaping.[33]

> As we build networks – patterns of synaptic patterns when very young, so we build the framework which will shape how we learn as we get older: such shaping will significantly determine what we learn – it will be both an opportunity, and a constraint. The broader and more diverse the experience when very young, the greater are the chances that, later in life, the individual will be able to handle open, ambiguous, uncertain and novel situations.

The early years of life are like the early years of moving into a new house. Whether you add an extension is dictated by life needs. How you allocate rooms, decorate rooms, heat rooms and organize furniture in rooms is dependent on how they will be used. As you become more settled, the urge to re-decorate, to extend, to build anew declines. You are now living in what has been built. All that an infant sees, hears, touches, smells or tastes shapes a connection at the synapse. The more the experience is repeated the more permanent the connection becomes. With experiences that are never or rarely occur, the connections never arrive or are never laid down. With insufficient electrical or chemical activity, proficiency in the second language, or an ear for perfect pitch, or an eye for artistic detail or a perfect left-footed pass never comes and eventually the possibility is gone forever.

Chapter **4**

Wired for desire:

the brain and the onset of puberty

This chapter contains the following sections:

⚕ **Brain development and adolescence**
The brain develops unevenly. Some areas of the brain develop earlier than others. More information about languages and co-ordination.

⚕ **Passion's slaves**
Why most adolescents, particularly boys, are not good at reading emotions. The sources of emotional response in the brain.

⚕ **Pay attention**
Attention – what it is, and how to get it and keep it. Two responses to threat. Why your mouth dries up just as you are about to give that talk.

⚕ **A forgotten secret of learning**
The brain circuitry of motivation and how it is linked with emotion. Why the best learning involves a degree of risk.

⚕ **Learning addicts**
The brain not only recognizes winning and losing, but also responds to the experience differentially. The brain can become 'addicted' to highs. What sort of highs?

... and will answer the following questions:

↦ What does brain science tell us about selection by ability at 11 years of age?

↦ Is it possible to teach emotional intelligence?

↦ Can I control my own fears? If so, how?

↦ What's the link between emotion and attention?

↦ How might learning become addictive?

Introduction

Picture the scene. You dare not go into the bedroom in daylight. You must not look at what is on the walls. Do not pick anything off the floor. Creep carefully, for it is asleep. Deep inside its nether regions a creature who was once your son/daughter lurks. It used to tidy its bedroom, it used to help with the shopping. Once upon a time it washed up. Now it has discovered mood swings! You have entered the adolescent bedroom. Hormones previously becalmed through childhood are suddenly raging with a vengeance. You pick up the tab.

If you are a parent of an adolescent, do not worry. Help, in the form of reassurance, has arrived. A growing body of research suggests that the mood swings, the antisocial behaviours, the tantrums and the sulks may not be exclusively hormonal but have their origin in pre-programmed changes in the adolescent brain. Three separate US studies attempt to map the development of the adolescent brain. The findings are of real significance for parents and a help for those educators who teach youngsters between the ages of 5 and 16.

Little is yet known about individual differences in the brain. Research tends to focus more on similarity than on difference. At some point in the future we will have adequate tools to give us differentiated profiles of children's learning potential, their learning dispositions and their thinking preferences. For the moment, we are a long way off. We do know, however, that differences exist and that some of those differences are in the maturation and development of the brain in and around the adolescent years.

Brain development and adolescence

Science points to a brain characterized by its uniqueness but we remain with a one-size-fits-all education system. Crucial choices influencing a child's future get made on the basis of chronological suitability, with the landmark choice moments occurring when the brain is at its most susceptible to change – around puberty. The brain, in its immature phases, develops not in a neat chronological continuum, but in spurts and plateaux, spurts and plateaux.

The pattern of spurts and plateaux varies by brain, and by function and region within the brain. At 11 years of age some parts of the country deem it expedient to make life-changing decisions about a child's learning potential based on paper and pencil tests notorious for measuring a narrow range of abilities. Brain profiling might allow similar decisions in the future to be timed by readiness rather than expedience. Brain profiling would lead us into a genuine education for inclusion.

Starting at about age 11, the brain undergoes major reorganization in areas associated with managing impulsivity, social interactions and risk evaluation. Debra Yurgelen Todd, Director of Neuroscience, Cognitive Psychology and Brian Imaging at the National Institute of Health, Boston, USA, is of the view that schools ought to pay more attention to the schooling of emotions, 'as important as teaching maths, science or reading is teaching social behaviours'. She points out that 'the neurobiology of development has not been systematically examined in healthy children and adolescents'. Her work looks specifically at the adolescent brain in development.[34]

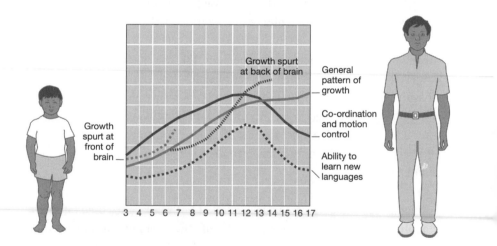

4.1 A growth spurt starts in the front of the brain from ages 3 to 6. Between 6 and 13, there is rapid growth towards the areas of the brain that are specialized for language skills. Growth rate areas of the brain linked to language are slow between the ages of 3 and 6 but speed up from 6 to 15. The ability to learn new languages declines rapidly after 12 years of age. Co-ordination ability declines in the brain from 13 to 15 when about 50 per cent of the brain tissue that controls motor skills are pruned away.

It has been assumed for many years that by the time a child began infant school all the hard-wiring had occurred and all that was left was for the programming of the system. Researchers presented a series of time-delayed images of developing brains from ages 3 through to 15.[35] The images show that the period around puberty is critical for the trimming of neural connections in the pre-frontal cortex. The pre-frontal cortex contributes to what are sometimes described as executive functions – evaluation of outcomes and of risk, impulse inhibition, interpretation of social cues – and is not fully developed until well after puberty. Adolescents in Yurgelen Todd's study were very poor at reading the emotions on the faces of individuals whose photographs they were shown. In many instances completely wrong interpretations were made: anger confused with joy; sadness with fear. Their brains had not yet been wired by experience of a range of social interactions.

In a project at Buffalo University 17 boys and 18 girls between the ages of 8 and 11 years were asked to perform two different types of face recognition tasks.[36] It was found that they used different parts of their brains to recognize faces and facial expressions. The boys used more of their right brain, while the girls used more of their left. Is it possible that the brains of males and females are organized differently before adulthood? This work suggests so.

For the first task, a face recognition memory task, the children had to identify 'target' faces that appeared on a series of slides. EEG equipment was used to measure electrical changes in the children's brain waves in the left and right hemispheres. The second task concentrated on identifying facial expressions from alternatives offered on a series of slides. This time there was no EEG measurement, but the researchers measured the accuracy and speed of the children's responses.

Although boys and girls were equally good at both tasks, they used different, though sometimes overlapping, parts of their brains to process the information. The researchers believe it is possible that boys process faces at a global level, an ability more associated with the right hemisphere of the brain. Conversely, girls may process faces at a more local level – an ability associated with the brain's left hemisphere. What if this were to be true? Would girls have an advantage in being better at 'reading' people and interpreting subtle changes in mood and behaviour?

On the west coast of the USA research being conducted at the same time found further valuable evidence that the adolescent brain develops in spurts and plateaux. Using MRI scans from children of normal health aged between 3 and 15 years, Dr Paul Thompson and his colleagues at UCLA found that children's brains develop in a specific pattern.[37] The researchers scanned the children's brains at intervals ranging from two weeks to four years, which allowed them to follow changes in their brains. The team detected striking, spatially complex patterns of growth and tissue loss. They identified a spurt of growth that starts in the front of the brain from ages three to six. Between the ages of 6 and 13, the researchers found that the pattern of rapid growth moves from the front to the back, towards the areas of the brain that are specialized for language skills. The researchers also found that growth rates in an area of the brain linked to language were slow between the ages of three and six but speeded up from 6 to 15 years when fine tuning of language usually occurs. The ability to learn new languages declines rapidly after the age of 12 years, as does the ability to recover language function if linguistic areas in one brain hemisphere are surgically resected.

A surprising finding for the Thompson team was that the brain did not grow at the same rate. Defying their expectations, they found that there are dynamic waves of growth in the brain. This leads them to believe that the most efficient time to learn a second language is in this period of growth.

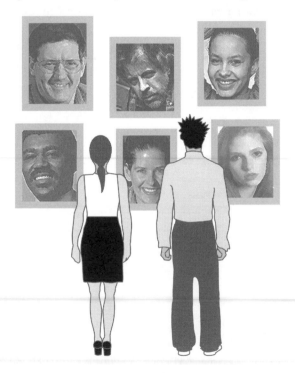

4.2 Is it possible that the brains of males and females are organized differently before adulthood? Work on face recognition showed that boys and girls use different parts of the brain when responding to different faces. Are girls 'naturally' better at reading people?

The UCLA team emphasize that the results are not meant to suggest that languages cannot be learned at older ages, but that 'it is simply a lot easier during those early pre-pubescent years'. Dr Thompson points out that these imaging results are supported by a number of surgical studies with patients suffering from brain injuries or tumours. These studies have shown that if the language cortex is removed before puberty, the brain is plastic enough to compensate for the loss. However, if the language cortex is removed after puberty, patients find it very difficult to reclaim their language skills.

The Thompson team also found that development of fine and large motor control, co-ordination of voluntary movement, began to decline in the brain from around age 13 to 15 when about 50 per cent of the brain tissue that controls motor skills are pruned away. Thus, activities that require motor skills, such as playing an instrument or a sport, may also have a critical period during childhood in which it is easiest to acquire the necessary abilities.

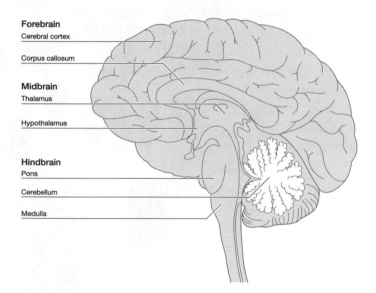

4.3   The major structures of the human brain showing forebrain, midbrain and brain stem. The brain is shown longitudinally with the front of the brain to the left. The major structures emerge from the spinal cord and include medulla, pons and cerebellum, all part of the brain stem. The midbrain contains the limbic and hippocampal areas. The forebrain, which is very prominent in humans, contains the cerebral cortex (which with the basal ganglia is called the cerebrum), the corpus callosum, thalamus and hypothalamus. The corpus callosum lies centrally between the right and left hemispheres and under the cerebral cortex.

The corpus callosum – 200 million nerve fibres going across a structure 10cm long and 2.5cm high – also completes its maturation in the late adolescent years. The corpus callosum acts like a relay station sending electrical signals between the two hemispheres of the cortex. Its successful development and integration is part of the wiring up of the adolescent brain. It is not considered to be fully integrated until the age range 16 through to about 25.

In a report produced for the UK-based ESRC,[38] authors Uta Frith and Sarah-Jayne Blakemore commented on the significance for educators of such research:

> These findings will need to be replicated and related to changes in learning. They may have implications for teaching. For instance, language learning and activities that require motor skills, such as playing an instrument or a sport, may have a critical period in which it is particularly easy to acquire these skills. Thus, brain imaging could in theory give a biological underpinning to concepts of critical/sensitive periods. In particular, it may be possible that research using diffusion tensor imaging will tell us about the development of myelination, connectivity, etc. and that this may relate to optimal windows for learning performance.

It is in the period to and around puberty that the emotional skills that will play such an important part in shaping our lives are being fine tuned. The frontal lobes will not be fully developed until late adolescence and early adulthood. The frontal lobes play an important part in emotional regulation. If you were to fail to develop the ability to recognize emotional responses in yourself and others, life will be hard for you.

Passion's slaves

Is it possible to develop emotional intelligence? Daniel Goleman authored a worldwide bestseller in his book *Emotional Intelligence: Why It Can Matter More Than IQ.*[39] He argues that a core set of emotional sensitivities can not only be identified but also be developed. This work is welcome, not for its understanding of the emotional circuitry of the brain, but because it opens a debate about identifying and developing a range of understandings appropriate to a wide variety of human experience. To attempt to measure emotional intelligence is a valuable endeavour but we are a long way off. This is nowhere near an exact science and never will be. The brain does not have one centre that runs all emotions. Emotional 'intelligence' presumes a correct response to certain situations, when in fact a variety of emotional responses could be valid. Emotional intelligence could become yet another exclusion measure if we are not careful. Harvard psychologist Jerome Kagan, whose child-development research Goleman uses to talk about the nature of shy and gregarious kids, warns that emotional intelligence has the same blindspots as IQ and some people 'handle anger well, but can't handle fear. Some people can't take joy.' Avoid the package. Recognize each emotion as distinct and plan for any intervention, if needed – and who is so well rounded they can decide? – with subtlety.

As a result of illness, a young English woman has recently had her amygdala removed in both hemispheres. The job of the amygdala is to alert us to dangerous, novel and interesting situations and to direct our internal readiness and reaction systems to respond appropriately. Fear and anger are two of four emotions that some cognitive psychologists believe make up the differently coloured threads from which is woven an emotional tapestry. This 'tapestry' you eventually settle on and retain for life: it is unique to the individual. The other emotions are joy and sadness. Some argue that surprise, disgust and guilt are aside from the basic four. Others argue that all other emotions are a mix from the original threads. What would your life become if you lost the ability to recognize and respond to basic emotions? Researchers at Cambridge University are monitoring her progress. She has no cognitive damage, she performs well on intellectual tests. She finds it impossible to recognize emotions and total difficulty recognizing fear and anger in other's voices. She has an intellectual understanding but no comprehension or ability to respond in real life.

The emotions determine what we give attention to. The emotions shape what is remembered and how it is remembered. The emotions dictate future behavioural response. Educators need a better understanding of the role of the emotions in human development. Too much of the prevailing models are dependent on common sense and on hearsay. A more informed understanding of the role of the emotions in learning and their manifestation in the brain will helps us design better learning models.

I grew up in a small town in Scotland in the 1960s and early 1970s. If you, like me, suffered badly from teenage angst, you will appreciate that a crucial part of that teenage angst was loyalty at a tribal level to certain types of music – even specific artistes. At that time it was commonplace to buy your clothing from the back pages of the *New Musical Express.* This journal specialized in flared denims called loons, often split at the knee and sometimes two-tone. It offered shirts in cheesecloth, kaftans and afghan coats. People who bought this journal and wore these clothes liked artistes such as Neil Young, Joni Mitchell and James Taylor. They smelled of joss-sticks and patchouli oil. I avoided them. I wore tartan shirts, braces, Levi's and boots that I bought from an emporium in the next town. I liked Slade and anything noisy. To this day I can sing the repertoire at the slightest hint of interest. To be honest, I can sing most of the other songs from that period too. If I do so, I am washed in nostalgia. The sights, smells, sounds, confused emotions and embarrassment become instantly real. Why?

I had always assumed I was 'passion's slave' except that my passions were rather banal. Now I discover that perhaps my brain, like that of every other adolescent, was altering in ways that actually made it better at remembering. The sights, smells, tastes, sounds and feelings of adolescence are encoded to make them more accessible years later. Work done on autobiographical memory and 'the lifetime retrieval curve' by Professor Martin Conway[40] describes 'the reminiscence bump'. The reminiscence bump occurs in the mid-teens and remains until the mid-twenties. In this phase of our lives we recall more memories. The shape of the bump is the same for different cultures although the type of memory varies and so does the timescale of the bump. In the United States the memories are more autonomous and more emotional. People remember more about their own experiences as individuals. Interestingly in China the memories tend to be more social. People remember whom they were with and the social setting. In the USA the earliest childhood memories tend to cluster around 40 months. In China it is nearer to 60 months. Memories differ because the prevailing culture shapes our concept of self. Who I am, is partly dependent on who I need to be. Different cultures assign different values on what success looks and feels like. Another reason we remember more around our formative years is that it is around this time that we wrestle with our concept of self. It is a highly emotional period.

Anything with a significant emotional resonance was being tagged for later recall. Experiences with a high level of emotional resonance are easier to recall than other memories. They remain unusually stable over time. This is because they have a completely different encoding and de-coding system. If you want to get something remembered, suffuse it with emotion.

The limbic system is a primitive centre deep within the brain that links the bodily response with the intellectual response. In this sense it takes primitive and instinctual drives and integrates those with the capacity to manage and make sense of those drives. It was first discussed by Dr Paul MacLean in 1967 when he also talked about three 'types' of brain.[41] MacLean argued that the brain's structures reflected its evolution and that we had kept the parts of our predecessor's brain that were of use. The 'reptilian' brain formed a control centre for everyday life where survival functions were monitored: respiration, heart rate, temperature control, automatic movement, arousal, rest. Sitting on top of this knob at the base of the brain was the limbic system, which co-ordinated survival responses and was responsible for emotional arousal and memory. Plonked on top once again was the neo-cortex, a late developer responsible for higher order functions such as planning and abstract thinking. Neuroscientists no longer talk in terms of 'triune' or three brains and have not done so for many years. The present generation of brain scientists may not even know what it means. Nor is the term limbic system used in the same way. However, for educators and others, they still offer a compelling metaphor for brain organization.

The limbic system includes anterior and posterior lobes. The anterior is actively engaged in emotional responses and the posterior with related memory and evaluation functions. It is, however, part of an integrated system so, for example, the memory of an experience can be 'state' dependent. Our recall improves when we are put back into that original state. To remember something really well, attach it to an emotional state. If there is too much emotion, then you get a dysfunctional response. If there is too little, then it is more difficult to retrieve. The development period to, and around, adolescence is a period of high emotional resonance. Something about the process of 'emotional tagging' makes it easier for recall.

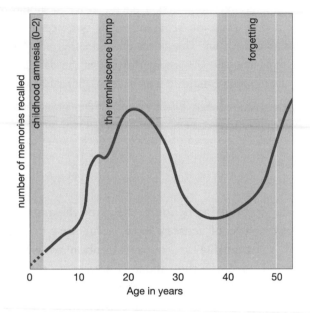

4.4 Autobiographical Memory and The Life Span Retrieval Curve. Our memories seem to be more distinct and more numerous around a period in our lives beginning just before puberty and for some years after.

There are many more pathways from the limbic system to cortex than the reverse. It seems we are designed to get information that has been emotionally 'tagged' as part of a response system. This may be part of the reason we react instinctively and before careful thought. This is the equivalent of taking the high road or the low road. Emotional 'tags' make that choice for you.

Pay attention

Sometimes we are so busy concentrating on the detail we do not notice the bigger changes. In an experiment at Harvard University, Professor Daniel J. Simons shows how we are often blind to change, especially if we are focused on detail.[42] At a library reception desk, students arrive to submit registration forms. When a desk assistant bends down he is a replaced by another, physically dissimilar, assistant. One bends down another pops up. Everything else remains as before and the assistant assumes the part his predecessor played. How many people noticed the change? Seventy-five per cent of Professor Simons's subjects did not notice the swap.

Dr Candace Pert says that the emotions help us decide what to remember and what to forget.

> In order for the brain not to be overwhelmed by the constant deluge of sensory input, some sort of filtering system must enable us to pay attention to what our bodymind deems the most important pieces of information and to ignore the others... Our emotions (or the psychoactive drugs that take over their receptors) decide what is worth paying attention to.[43]

If the students had been involved in some sort of emotional tryst with one or other of the receptionists, you can bet they would have noticed the change. If, the day before, they had a blazing row with one of them, they would have noticed. Remove emotional resonance and we are in the land of the bland. Attention and recall systems are affected by emotion.

The high road choice involves a different set of systems from the low road choice. The high road involves a 'relatively slow, analytic, reflective (primarily cortical) system to explore the objective, factual elements of a situation, to compare them with related memories of past experience, and then to rationally respond'.[44] The high road system is useless in an emergency. It will not get you in trouble but sometimes, when an immediate response is required, it will not get you out of it either.

The low road choice is more primitive, more survival focused and more likely to bypass analysis and higher order considerations. It is shaped by instinct and primed by basic emotion. It is the rapid response system experienced when confronted by a predator. It is a whole body response, fast but exhausting. It gets you away from immediate danger. The high road choice is reflective. The low road choice is reflexive. One is slow, the other fast. Your low road or reflexive system is also the default mode: 'In confusion go to this', 'If uncertain, or in data overload, activate low road response.' Going to default is what happens when you metaphorically 'see red'. With a 'sudden rush of blood to the head' you respond through a learned behaviour acquired in a formative phase. For example, you are a car driver. When you learned to drive the car the horn was in the centre of the steering column. Years later you are in a different car with the horn down by the side of the steering column. Someone cuts you up at a junction. What do you do? In a sudden rage you may find yourself beating the centre of the steering column with the flat of your hand or, worse, you give him a quick flick of your windscreen washers! Why? Learned behaviours or default behaviours assert themselves when you are stressed.

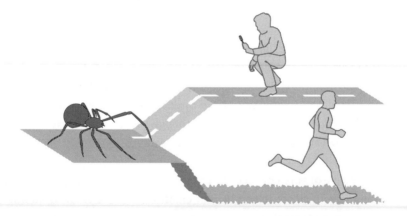

4.5 High and low road responses to everyday stimulus. The response to the spider differs if you are a collector or if you are a phobic. One is a high road response and the other a low road response. Is education about increasing the high road choices available to our children?

Fear always evokes a low road response. Some children have a fear of school. It is really difficult to remove conditioned fears once we have learned to be afraid of something. Again, there are good survival reasons for this.

There is a biological basis to most phobias. Many others are learned responses from which it has become difficult to break. Good survival-oriented phobias include the fear of anything that might pose danger: open spaces where predators proliferate; closed spaces where escape from predators is impossible: shapes that seem to slither or crawl; creatures that leap at you; objects that may fall on you; objects that you may fall off; things that brush your face and threaten your air passages.

All these experiences are potentially low road. It happens and you mobilize. For example, you visit the zoo. With your two young children you go to the reptile house to see what is there. For some reason it is cool, damp and gloomy. Not a good start. As you stand, separated from the 2cm of bullet-proof plate glass by a rope attached to bollards, you notice that on the other side of the glass a lizard-like thing of some size is having lunch. Lunch is being dropped in and, as it eats, there is a lot of tugging and wrenching near the glass. So three of you watch transfixed and separated by bollards, rope, 60cm of space and 2cm of plate glass. Your mind wanders into reverie at the point when, catching a glimpse of itself reflected by your dark sweater against the glass and fearing a rival, the lizard pounces only to be stopped by the glass wall. What is your response? Is it high or low road? High road would be, 'Ooh I wonder if it poses any sort of threat? What do you think children?' Low road does not involve any conscious thought, it is a leap backwards with a gulp of breath and your hands brought to readiness to defend yourself.

The difference explains how the system works to our advantage. More and more, neuroscientists are telling us that emotions are 'the result of multiple brain and body systems that are distributed over the whole person', and that 'we cannot separate emotion from cognition or cognition from the body.'[45] Motor and emotion systems are in close proximity within the brain. The emotions are expressed throughout the body in physiological changes, some of which are subtle and many others, like the survival responses, less so. Some are learned – a disparaging frown, for instance – and some are hard-wired into the brain: laughter, blushing, smiling and the startle response.

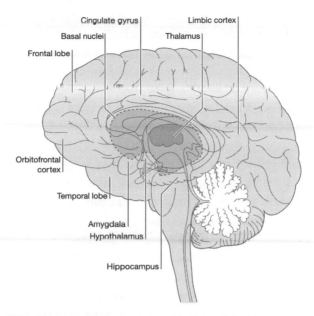

4.6   The amygdala is close to and in front of the hippocampus.
Shown in cross section to illustrate proximity to the frontal
lobes. There are more connections from the limbic system
including the amygdala up into the cortex than the reverse,
and more connections from the frontal lobes into the
amygdala than from any other part of the brain.

The mechanics of high and low road response systems tells us about emotion
and learning. To understand human motivation, you need to know about the
limbic system and, more specifically, the amygdala. It could be described as
the 'Trojan mouse' of motivation: upon this small site, all else depends. It
plays a powerful part in labelling or tagging something as 'significant'. When
an experience has been 'tagged', we respond thereafter in very different
ways.

The amygdala is a part of the limbic system that we described above. It is very
small, the size of your thumb nail, and is almond shaped. There are a dozen
or so neural clusters comprising the amygdala. Each of these clusters links
with different structures elsewhere in the brain and utilizes different
chemical messengers to facilitate connections. The amygdala is involved in
regulation of arousal, sleep, immune systems, movement, reproduction and
memory. The amygdala seems particularly involved in aggression, fear and
fear's younger brother and sister, anxiety and worry. The amygdala's closest

friends are the frontal lobes. The frontal lobes are involved in managing impulsivity, long-term planning, discrimination and fine judgement, and goal-setting. The amygdala and the frontal lobes seem to hang out together; they have good connections. There are more connections from the limbic system including the amygdala up into the cortex than the reverse, and there are more connections from the frontal lobes into the amygdala than from any other part of the brain. The two are an act.

Imagine you find yourself in a novel situation that has, for you, an element of threat. The threat is not real. It is not life threatening, but it has the modern-day equivalence. You are on a training course and you are going to be asked to speak. What happens?

From the amygdala, communications go two ways. The first goes direct to the senses and to the thalamus. The thalamus is a structure in the brain that traffics sensory information such as vision, hearing and touch. You go on alert. The second goes to the internal response system via the hypothalamus. At the same time, whoosh, the amygdala sends information direct to the brain stem, which regulates breathing, heart rate, body temperature, blood pressure. At the thought of having to talk in front of your peers your amygdala has gone on red alert!

Your response has an internal and external aspect initiated at first through the same system. Internally adrenaline starts to flow, blood pressure rises, breathing gets faster, heart rate goes up and you are mobilized for response. Externally you blush, your body posture stiffens, you become more fidgety and you perspire. Now if there is a previous embarrassing experience of speaking that has been tagged as such, then this happens more quickly. What happens is another brain structure known as the basal nuclei gets a message from its near neighbour in the limbic system, the amygdala, that something out of the ordinary is going on and it gets involved. One of the things it does is release a chemical messenger up into the cortex called acetylcholine. This guarantees that this experience will get remembered in the future. The chemical speeds up the firing pattern between neurons and the system moves to overload. You get a sinking feeling in your gut and your mouth feels dry.

A forgotten secret of learning

Motivation has been described as a 'process that ties emotion to action' – emotion in motion. The word motivate has Latin origins and means 'to move' This is the same origin as e-motion. My simple contention would be that motion and e-motion are two forgotten secrets of learning. In experiencing motivation many levels of the brain become involved. According to Danah Zohar, a leading researcher into spirituality and the brain, 'the human brain rewires itself when it is interested, passionate and creative'.[46] Motivate yourself and your brain responds accordingly.

High road and low road systems are involved when we experience true motivation. How quickly might you react if your child was about to cross a busy street with a car only metres away and closing fast? You cannot answer. The speed of your low road, reflexive response system would astonish you. To be properly motivated we need to be able to tag an experience or a prospect with a strong enough tag. For the tag to have value to us at high and low levels, it must have an emotional significance. I always tell teachers to sell benefits not features to their students, and sell those benefits at the personal level. By doing this you engage the extended amygdala. This is your route to the primary pleasure centre.

Research into human brains and reward learning is a growing field. Work has been done in addiction research and also into the effect of the brain on perceived financial reward.[47] In animal research, the dopamine reward systems, which include the amygdala, basal ganglia and pre-frontal cortex, are all involved when animals are 'bribed' by food or, indeed, with mild drugs. Research done with monkeys by Michael Merzenich showed how connections between brain cells were dramatically enhanced when a reward system was built into a task. On the cortex there are regions of the brain responsible for touch. Using scanning technology, the cells were mapped as the monkeys played with a slowly revolving wheel. Then Merzenich added an incentive. When the monkeys responded to a pattern and speed of spinning and pressed a buzzer, they were rewarded with food. As they became expert, the neurons devoted to recall of the task proliferated. Neural networks close by were also recruited. The incentive had played its part in enhancing the recall. It mattered to the monkey therefore it was tagged as significant, neural investment was made and the process was remembered. Proof positive that motivation matters in learning.

The cingulate gyrus is the main link thereafter: it is the main conduit between motivation and reward. It has the sensory mechanisms to receive processed visual, auditory, kinesthetic, gustatory and olfactory information while also getting information about the internal readiness of the body. As it assembles the information, it sends it off to different areas of the brain. Thus, the basal ganglia is contacted for motor reaction, the brain stem for physiological arousal and the hippocampus for appropriate memory.

Prompted by the amygdala, the cingulate gyrus is the main conduit between emotion and reward. It is taking in data about levels of physical readiness, arousal and past experience and then, on the basis of this tagging, as significant or otherwise. Thus decisions get made very quickly about appropriate levels of response.

The amygdala and cingulate gyrus will be actively involved in learning that is meaningful. Meaningful learning engages powerful emotions because it involves risk. What appears to a skilled learner to be mundane – 'Will I get this wrong?' – can for others be highly intimidating. Ask yourself the question, 'What do I remember most distinctly about school?' I guess that, in the main, your recollections may be positive. Could this indicate that you had successes there? To be interested in, and (still) reading, this book shows a level of comfort with things academic. This is not necessarily shared by the majority of the population. When I ask public audiences 'What do you remember most distinctly about school?', the overwhelming, and sad, response is negative. Adults talk at length about being humiliated, being intimidated, being overlooked or forgotten. In formal learning why would a learner take the risk of saying 'I don't know' if the consequence is humiliation, intimidation or neglect? Participating in a formal learning environment is like a visit to life's bookmaker. You have to make the choice of going for the big money. It needs a large personal stake. You risk losing and the losses will be emotional, not financial, and the scars will remain. Those in whom we can develop the healthy risk taking that is meaningful learning become hooked for life. Those who take a big loss early on do not come back in the shop. How can we make sense of risk-taking behaviour?

There are three motivators for taking on risk. If a benefit is self-evident or made to appear so, if we can connect to that benefit at a personal level and feel that its achievement is possible, then we may take the risk of going for it. The thinking that accompanies this process is one where we switch from present to future and back again – future to present – again and again. If we can make the desired outcome bigger, brighter and more attractive, it may become compelling enough for us to move from the present. The present position has attractions of certainty and security. If it can be made uncertain, insecure and sufficiently unattractive, then we will also feel compelled to move. The movement itself may carry enough promise for us to do it anyway. We may carry memories of similar risks that are pleasurable enough to want us to revisit. The behaviours may themselves generate a vague pleasurable state that is enough for their reinforcement. So we have three motivators for risk: a compelling future, an undesirable present or a vague pleasure in the experience itself.

Learning addicts

Scientists such as Antonio Damasio have shown that the frontal areas of the brain, and specifically the ventral pre-frontal regions, may be an important link between intellectualizing risk and how one 'feels' about risk.[48] Gamblers who have damage to these areas of the brain do not exhibit any appreciation of the three possible responses and remain locked in pleasure seeking.

Gambling changes hormone levels in the body. If this is so, then gambling could be classed as an addiction. Heart rates and cortisol levels were higher in gamblers playing with their own money than playing for points. A team from the University of Bremen studied the physical changes that took place in men playing blackjack. The gamblers reported feeling surges of euphoria when they placed bets. Dr Gerhard Meyer suggests that this echoes the euphoria experienced by drug takers, which results from a surge of the neurotransmitters dopamine and serotonin in the brain: 'The theory behind addiction is that if you consume an [addictive] substance, more dopamine is released than normal, and this is what happens when people consume drugs or alcohol. When people gamble, they say they feel this euphoria through a behavioural surrogate. Cortisol may contribute to such mood alterations.'[49] In a similar experiment, neural responses to reward were measured while gamblers played poker.[50] This time they played for money and the scientists compared brain activity to how well the poker players were doing. If a player lost, the hippocampus was more active. If a player won, the midbrain became more active. As a player won more and more, the pleasure centres in the brain became more active. This included centres associated with control of movement, with control of excitement and higher thought. If a player happened to lose more and more, there were very different responses in these same brain areas. At the time of writing, there is research taking place with individuals who are addicted to shopping. They are a self-selecting group who volunteered – in part – as a way of overcoming credit card problems. The outcomes are awaited with interest (at 2.3 per cent above base over a 12-month period).

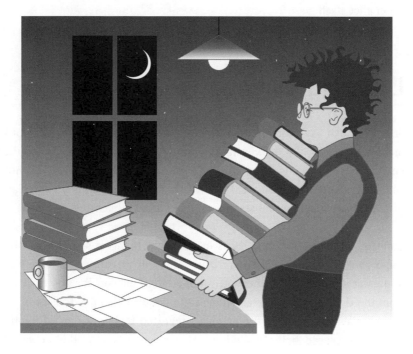

4.7 The brain responds differentially to the thought of winning. Many schools focus on failure and many learners in those schools opt out from the gamble of learning. They expect failure. Should we do more in our schools to sell the benefits? Can we create a generation of learning addicts?

So what? This work shows that the brain not only recognizes winning and losing, but it also responds to the experience differentially and in a way that is dependent on the advantage or disadvantage experienced. If it is possible to get a high from gambling, why should it not be possible to get a high from learning? Is the absence of a learning high in the schooling of 99.9 per cent of the population because they are never persuaded to take real risks. When learning is passive, it does not engage any sort of emotion other than perhaps apathy. When it is individualized and has an emotional resonance, then we get dopamine learning and it sticks. We become addicted to the high that is negotiating and overcoming personal risk. Reinforce it enough and we get learning addicts.

The nucleus accumbens also works by tagging information that has a positive emotional signal. It is a 'pleasure seeker' sited deep within the brain. It can be aroused to action very quickly and it remembers. It says to itself and to other areas of the brain, 'I enjoyed this, I'd like to enjoy it again...' It too is linked to the amygdala. Heavy smokers activate the nucleus accumbens every time they light up. If you stimulate the nucleus accumbens of rats, it helps them learn more quickly. Tag the experience with pleasure! A child who suffers from a deficiency in the brain's reward system may over-compensate by indulging in substances or behaviours that are in themselves rewarding. Reward deficiency syndrome states that a lack of internal rewards leads a person to 'self-medicate' in this way.

Curiously enough some researchers would say that apathy seems to be a specific malfunction of the motivation circuits of the brain. It is a neurological condition masked by other related problems. I would like to go into this in more detail, but it will have to wait until I can get around to it!

Joseph Le Doux says that at the neural level, 'each emotional input consists of a set of inputs, an appraisal mechanism and a set of outputs'.[51] The appraisal mechanisms are either programmed by nature – 'natural triggers' – or are acquired through experience – 'learned triggers'. Triggers can be positive or negative – and all shades in between – with different neural systems devoted to them. Hence, there is no emotional brain but a series of emotional response systems. Antonio Damasio suggests that people learn appropriate emotional responses through everyday experience.[52] Then the decision-making process about behavioural responses is facilitated by a 'somatic marker' that narrows the range of alternatives. When working well this means that we can read facial expressions, body language, contextual cues and operate good choices. If there is damage to the pre-cortical region of your brain, you may be less skilled at making choices. Patients with damage to this area – including the gamblers – had flatter emotional ranges and were prone to making bad life choices because they were no longer guided by their emotions. Both Le Doux and Damasio suggest that conscious thought is primed by an underlying emotional sensing. This can occur outside of conscious awareness. Intuition nudges the choices we make. In the next chapter we will find out more about intuition and learning.

Chapter **5**

Wired to inspire:

the completion of brain development

This chapter contains the following sections:

⍏ Thinking is hard work
Thinking burns energy. When we think, different neural structures are called on to assist. Knowing which neural structures can help in learning design.

⍏ The tuition of intuition
Thinking independently is not a given. Much of our thinking is determined by factors outside of conscious awareness. Intuition, an integral part of creativity, is foreclosed by Western education.

⍏ Mathematics and the brain
Two types of mathematical thinking exposed by brain scientists. Why they may have great value for maths teachers.

⍏ We are all musical!
Science proves we all have musical ability. How music can aid learning. Why Mozart will not make you a better thinker.

⍏ Doing 'Good Looking'
Developing the ability to 'look' with different parts of the brain. Using visual stimuli better in classrooms.

⍏ Mental rehearsals of success
The proof that you can develop muscles by thought. How to develop the mental rehearsal muscles of children.

... and will answer the following questions:

▷ Does thinking tire you out?

▷ Can I learn something without being aware that I am doing so?

▷ How do I help my child improve at maths?

▷ Why are some people more musically gifted than others?

▷ Does a trained artist look at a painting with the same parts of the brain as an amateur?

▷ Can I improve my performance in a sport just by thinking about it?

Introduction

What is going on in your brain when you learn to play the piano or when you learn to read or practise maths or learn to paint? Is there a part of the brain for algebra and a separate part for geometry? Do you use different parts of the brain for learning a foreign language? What about different parts of the brain for different languages? One of the most exciting possibilities offered to educators by neuroscience is the hope that soon we will not only be able to identify how the brain is used for specific learning functions but also be able to modify and improve the brain structures used. It is highly unlikely that the sort of intellectual engagement required by one discipline activates the same neural structures as a different discipline. The sort of thinking required for artistic creativity is not the same as algebraic calculation. So what do we know about the different sorts of thinking and brain activity?

According to Professor Robert Sternberg the essence of intelligent thought would 'seem to be in knowing when to act quickly, and knowing when to think and act slowly'.[53] Is there a best way to think? If so, can it be taught? We are often advised to think 'hard about it' or give it 'serious thought'. But what might thinking hard mean? What happens in the brain? Is thinking tiring? Can thinking hard actually cause fatigue?

Thinking is hard work

I was recently told a story about a group of young people spending a weekend on a residential course in practical thinking and problem solving. It was to be run and organized by the British Army and would take place on Dartmoor, a secluded expanse of moorland in south-west England. The students, all around the ages of 12 to 14, were to be helped to develop their thinking skills in an environment that would also prove challenging. They were from city areas and did not have much knowledge of any locality other than their own backyard. They were asked to bring with them a packed lunch of some sort for day one. The hosts would provide all the other meals. One boy, a likeable lad from a disadvantaged background, arrived with a brown paper bag. This contained his lunch. As lunchtime arrived he looked perplexed and miserable. The others were tucking in to sandwiches, cakes and crisps. He did not know how to begin to eat his lunch, which turned out to be two uncooked potatoes still covered in earth.

A team from the University of Virginia in the USA carried out research on rats and how thinking consumes energy.[54] They found that having to 'think harder' drains glucose from a key part of the brain. The effect was more dramatic in older rats, whose brains also took longer to recover. Dr Ewan McNay said, 'The brain runs on glucose. Young rats can do a pretty good job of supplying all the glucose that a particular area of the brain needs until a task demanding that brain area becomes difficult. In older rats, even on tasks that cause no glucose drainage in young rats, we see big problems in supplying the brain with glucose. This correlates with a big deficit in performance. A lack of fuel affects the ability to think and remember.' If the young lad out on the moors is not able to convert his two potatoes into some form of nutrition, then his capacity to think, already limited it would seem, is going to be drastically curtailed.

One of the implications of this research is that the contents and timing of meals may need to be co-ordinated to have the most beneficial effects to enhance thinking and learning. Those who set up breakfast clubs in schools help overcome some of the process of metabolic starvation brought on by poor fuelling habits.

Glucose is the main source of energy for the brain. It has long been thought that, unless a person is starving, the brain always receives an ample supply of glucose. The Virginia team measured glucose levels in the brains of rats as they navigated their way through a maze. They found that in a brain area concerned with visual and spatial memory the demand for glucose was so high that levels fell by 30 per cent. However, levels stayed constant in other brain areas that played no role in spatial memory.

In a follow up study, the researchers showed that in older rats glucose levels in the active brain areas dropped by 48 per cent during the maze task. They also found that in the older animals glucose supply did not return to normal until 30 minutes after the task was completed. In young rats recovery was immediate.

The researchers found they could boost the performance of the rats by giving them glucose injections. Professor David Gold said, 'Glucose enhances learning and memory not only in rats but also in many populations of humans. For schoolchildren, this research implies that the contents and timing of meals may need to be co-ordinated to have the most beneficial effects that enhance learning.'

Would playing a game such as chess exercise and thus develop the brain? If so, what structures in the brain would benefit? If you are about to checkmate an opponent, you are working hard and doing so against the clock. All knowledge and experience is brought to the moment. You are perceiving colours, shapes and combinations of possible moves on the board and separating these out from activity in the periphery of your senses. You are assigning value to the pieces. You retrieve the rules. You consider consequences and recognize and retrieve familiar patterns. Your mind shifts between reflection and speculation, back and forward, back and forward.

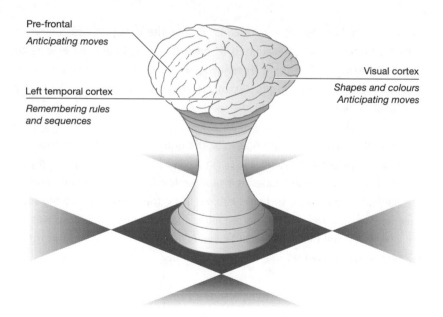

Pre-frontal
Anticipating moves

Visual cortex
Shapes and colours
Anticipating moves

Left temporal cortex
Remembering rules
and sequences

5.1 Thinking reorganizes the brain. Thinking can be locally and globally focused. Both types of thinking are desirable. Chess players exhibit both. Visual processing centred at the back of the brain identifies shapes and colours. Structures in the left temporal cortex are used for remembering rules and sequences of moves. Anticipating moves activates both pre-frontal and visual cortex.

In a 1994 research project ten chess players played each other under competition conditions while being monitored by Positron Emission Tomography (PET) – a method for detecting chemical changes within the brain.[55] It was found that glucose uptake was raised in very different neural structures simultaneously. This suggested that the brain was 'working hard' to perform the game. Separating colours and identifying shapes activated parts on both sides of the brain towards the back of the head known to be associated with visual processing. Remembering the rules and 'sequences of plays' activated two parts on the left side of the brain, a small structure deep within the brain associated with indexing memories and a structure in an area near the left ear associated with memory storage. Forward planning and, specifically, 'checkmate' activated both the pre-frontal cortex (vital for planning and fine judgement) and the visual cortex (for mental rehearsal of the look of the moves).

Structured intellectual activity such as chess offers the player an opportunity to integrate very different functional specialisms within the brain in an experience shared with others. It also requires the successful practitioner to think globally and locally simultaneously. You must focus on the move but not lose sight of the chain of consequences. As such, it provides a cameo of some sound learning principles: simultaneous global and local thinking, reflection and speculation, structured challenge, agreed measures of performance, shared experience upon which to draw, open-ended outcomes.

The tuition of intuition

Can you think without being aware of doing so? Is effort a necessary part of thinking? If we can have intuitive knowledge, does this mean that we can learn without awareness?

Our unconscious thought processes support conscious thought. When I lift the cup to my mouth I do not have to attend to the separate movements of all the muscles in my right hand and arm, nor do I have to look at the cup to guide it safely to my mouth, nor do I have to take deliberate care to open my mouth before I start to drink. After initiating the process, there is little conscious decision making involved. At a level outside of conscious awareness behaviours are being initiated. Such behaviours have been learned and then rehearsed over time. They are now part of me. What other behavioural responses of which I am no longer consciously aware might be part of me?

Repeated exposure to phenomena develops a favourable view of it even if we do not consciously seek that view. This is known as 'positive effect'. Independently of what I want at a conscious level my thinking is being shaped by 'familiarity'. Research conducted with fake words and with photographs of people's faces showed that when asked to rank the fake words or the faces in terms such as 'which word might best mean "goodness"?' or, 'which face do you like the most?' control groups favoured those that they had seen more often. In both cases and again and again, there was a strong correlation between frequency of exposure and positive effect. The more the control groups had seen the fake words or the photograph, the more they were attracted to it. This means that much of our thinking is determined or primed by familiarity. Thought is not so independent as we might think!

In learning it is possible through participating in an activity to 'learn' embedded rules and codes of conduct without being consciously aware of doing so. If you have a telephone number with ten or more digits, you will tend to remember it in chunks. This is effective to such a degree that if you buy something over the phone and the vendor repeats back your telephone number, you may not recognize it immediately if the vendor is chunking it differently. At no time have you consciously sat down and practised your telephone number. It has been assimilated through exposure.

Research on implicit learning shows you have capability of learning procedures, rules, patterns of 'play' and complex sequences without focused attention on doing so. When the pattern of brain activation is mapped in games players practising a simple reaction time task, changes occur. Without being consciously aware of any pattern embedded in what they were asked to do, the players rehearsed the reaction time task again and again. There was, in fact, a complex sequence hidden within the activity. After extended rehearsal, a very slight alteration in the sequence of the game resulted in immediate and corresponding blood flow changes in the brain. There was more activity in the left pre-motor area, left anterior cingulate, and right ventral striatum. Activation was reduced in the right dorsolateral pre-frontal and parietal areas. Without the games players being aware of it, learning had occurred. The brain had become more efficient at dealing with the embedded pattern. The researchers believe that the ventral striatum is responsive to new information, and the right pre-frontal area is associated with the maintenance of known information. They also believe that you can conduct an activity that simultaneously requires understanding context and developing new skills without being consciously aware of doing so.

Schools are good at doing bits of information. They are not so good at the joins. The Western curriculum tends to be packaged up in discrete bits attended to for given periods of time within a recognized chronological window. The brain is better at doing connections than doing bits and will, without the conscious engagement of its owner, seek to find connections. Albert Einstein noted that 'the relationship between two entities is more important than the entities themselves'. If we are connection seekers, if we seek the connections consciously and unconsciously, and if conscious seeking is the exception rather than the rule, we ought to be acutely self-conscious about the embedded learning that occurs on an everyday basis within and without our classrooms. Learning itself is all about seeking and securing connections. Finding and looking after the joins is what schools should be doing. At the synapse, the more cells that fire together, the more secure the connections thereafter.

Mathematics and the brain

Dyscalculia, or difficulty with numbers, affects between 3 per cent and 6 per cent of the population in the West. The trauma is as painful as that experienced by dyslexics. Imagine being unable to work out change, tell the time or catch the correct bus. Maths involves symbols as well as letters, and a plus sign + looks very similar to the letter x for many people. The language of maths is also potentially confusing, and if young learners latch onto the first interpretation of a phrase or word, then 'take-away' remains somewhere you get your Chinese food from on a Saturday night. Professor Brian Butterworth of University College London, author of *The Mathematical Brain* (2000), has shown that dyscalculic children are troubled by even the simplest numerical tasks such as selecting the larger of two numbers or counting the number of objects in a display. His research suggests there is a genetic basis for the problem. The next time you hear someone say 'I'm no good at maths – I get it from my dad' there might be a grain of truth in it. He also suggests that in some cases it arises as a result of bad teaching. If you are taught in a way that leaves flawed understanding and then you are asked to move on and build on top of the flawed understanding, it can lead to alienation.

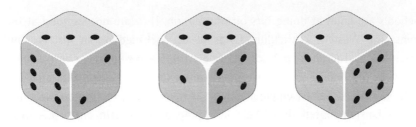

5.2 What is the total on the three dice? How did you arrive at the total? Did you add the dots? Did you also have to count the dice? We all add the dots. We do not count the dice.

Some of the world's leading researchers into mathematical thinking believe that infants display a sense of number. They can count, do elementary addition and subtraction and have an understanding of relationships in number. What is more, many animals show the same abilities! Professor Butterworth maintains that the brain has evolved special circuits for numbers, and maths is built on a 'specific innate basis whereas reading is not'.[56] Although the specialists would say that work on dyscalculia is about 20 years behind that on dyslexia, development of diagnostic tests for dyscalculia is in place and they should be available to educators soon.

A dyscalculic child would be more likely to:

- show difficulty in learning simple number concepts.
- have impaired sense of number size
- be poor at estimation.
- have problems navigating up and down number lines especially in 2s, 3s or more.

- find difficulty with new terms – for example, units in tens, hundreds or thousands.

- have difficulty linking facts to procedures – for example, subtract 2 from 7.

- show functional impairment of the parietal lobe.

- have 'normal' cognitive and language abilities but occasionally have other masking learning difficulties.

How does the brain deal with different types of mathematical reasoning? Some recent research might help improve the teaching of dyscalculic children. A team of French and American researchers were led by cognitive neuroscientist Stansilaus Dehaene of the National Institute of Health and Medical Research in Paris and cognitive psychologist Elizabeth Spelke of the Massachusetts Institute of Technology.[57] They say they have established that two very different brain functions are involved.

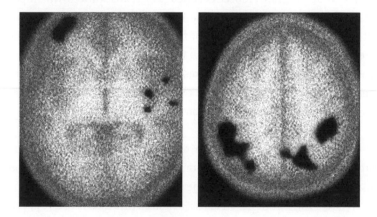

5.3   The scan on the left shows how the left frontal lobe, an area of the brain known to make associations between words, lit up when subjects were asked to make exact calculations. Estimation involved the left and right parietal areas.

Previous studies of brain-damaged patients have hinted that different areas may be used for different mathematical activities. One is a non-verbal, visual and spatial sense of quantity, the other has to do with symbols related to language. Mathematicians themselves have suggested that this might be so.

Albert Einstein said numerical ideas came to him more or less as images that he could combine at will, whereas others have said they rely on verbal representations of numbers when thinking about problems.

Volunteers who were fluent in two languages – English and Russian – were asked to solve a series of problems after first being taught the necessary maths. One group was taught in Russian, the other in English. The first thing to be discovered was that exact calculation needed more time. If they learned in English and were tested in Russian or vice versa, they needed as much as a second more to calculate exactly. Does 53 plus 68 equal 121 or 127? When they were tested on approximation – is 53 plus 68 closer to 120 or 150? – there was no time delay. The brain appears to be solving the tasks in two very different ways. Despite the seeming similarity of the tasks the difference was marked.

The volunteers were then tested in more complex mathematical operations, such as addition in a base other than 10 and the approximation of logarithms and square roots. The difference remained. PET scans showed which parts of the brain were operating in each kind of task. Exact calculations lit up the volunteers' left frontal lobe, an area of the brain known to make associations between words. Estimation involved the left and right parietal lobes – responsible for visual and spatial representations. The parietal lobes are also responsible for finger control – and counting on the fingers is something children almost everywhere do early on in learning exact arithmetic.

Explaining the findings, Dr Dehaene pointed out that many studies have indicated that the impact of education is probably much greater than any initial difference in innate ability. The findings will not, therefore, predict which children will naturally be better at maths. However, the results could lead to improved teaching methods. A practical idea would be to encourage children to talk themselves and others through their workings more frequently. Teachers should make every effort to use visual and spatial representations as well as oral explanations when teaching maths.

In the adult, imaging studies how the intraparietal area, located in the brain above each ear, and which is involved in visuo-spatial processing, is the area of the brain for 'number sense'. Damage to this area leads to dyscalculia. Dr Dehaene is of the view that the parietal lobe is actively involved in our ability to make sense of number from the earliest.[58] As we engage with the world of numbers and experience schooling, the non-verbal representation system known as the quantity system is repeatedly linked to other systems for numbers that are visual – symbols – or verbal – words – or both. Rote is predominantly verbal. Approximation is predominantly quantity. What would happen if there was an impairment in areas of the brain used to service quantity, visuo-spatial or verbal systems? When this happens we have difficulty with numbers. A genetic weakness could lead to a problem. So could a disorder arising from brain trauma. In a less obvious way, if there is poor development in neural structures connecting the processing areas, there may be loss of fluency. If I am over reliant on one strategy, then I could suffer as a consequence. Learning multiplication tables by rote is fine but not if I am unable to connect each outcome to a sense of quantity.

Brian Butterworth (2000) confirms that the brain uses different memory systems for the storage of mathematical information – including facts and procedures – to that used for ordinary 'everyday' information. Declarative and procedural memories rely on the temporal and frontal lobes. Maths facts and procedures seem more reliant on the parietal lobe. So, as we have seen, any damage to this area has a profound impact. It is vital for maths teachers to help children understand the process of what they are doing. Learning number patterns by rote is like learning a narrative poem: it activates language and not number centres in the brain. Knowing facts does not necessarily make you better at manipulating number systems. Knowing how to manipulate number systems makes you better with number facts. It seems there is a neurological basis for this distinction. In addition to practice in manipulating numbers, articulating the methodology behind it is important. Reflective rehearsal allows the maths procedures to be stored in long-term memory. Reflectivity thus leads to reflexive responses. The more you do it in a considered way and have opportunities to reflect on doing so, the more of a reflex it becomes. Next time, you go there automatically. It has been learned.

One scientist entered the dangerous field of explaining the effect of technology on a child's brain by suggesting that computer games are damaging to brain development. Professor Ryuta Kawashima and his team at Tohoku University in Japan compared the brain activity of children playing Nintendo with children doing a simple, repetitive mental arithmetic exercise.

The team claimed that the game stimulated those parts of the brain associated with vision and with movement whereas the arithmetic stimulated activity in both left and right hemispheres of the frontal lobe. Kawashima took the unusual step, for a neuroscientist, of making a judgement about the ideal learning conditions as a result of his findings. 'There is a problem we will have with a new generation of children who play computer games that we have never seen before. The implications are very serious for an increasingly violent society and these students will be doing more and more bad things if they are playing games and not doing other things like reading aloud or learning arithmetic'.[59]

We are all musical!

Should you wish to, you can buy a boxed set of CDs entitled *Baroque a Bye Baby*. It includes classical pieces that the publishers claim will develop your baby's brain. Simply tuck in the child, turn up the volume and away you go – neural structures activated aplenty! How useful a practice might this be? Is there any way in which playing classical pieces of music to very young children enhances their capacity for learning? Is there such a thing as a Mozart effect? Is there any benefit to the brain in learning to play a musical instrument? If so, what instrument, to what level and when should a child start to learn? If I am a musician, how is my brain different from my nextdoor neighbour's?

According to Professor Gordon Shaw of USC Irvine and co-originator of the 'Mozart effect' research, 'training a child in music at three or four years of age improves the way in which their brain recognizes pattern in space and time'.[60] There is a great deal of accumulated evidence of the all-round advantages of an early training in music. To follow a discipline of smooth, controlled, voluntary, cross-lateral movement, with both hands - and possibly feet - involved and simultaneously tracking the notes on a page so as to anticipate the sounds to come is a great all-round work-out for the brain. To do so regularly and for pleasure is a wonderful thing. Some would have us believe it makes you more intelligent. Professor Norman Weinberger is of the view that 'millions of neurons can be activated in a single musical experience'.[61] He adds, 'music has an uncanny manner of activating neurons for purposes of relaxing muscle tension, changing pulse and producing long-range memories which are directly related to the number of neurons activated in the experience.' Music offers educators the possibility of energizing or relaxing students, carrying content information, priming certain types of cognitive performance and enhancing phonological awareness.

What is the Mozart effect? The Mozart effect is a term which has been corrupted through a game of global Chinese whispers. Work done by Professor Shaw and his team found that 'undergraduates in a control group undertaking mathematical tasks involving spatial and rotational symmetry, showed significant performance improvements when played a Mozart Piano Sonata for two Pianos in D for 10 minutes prior to the task'. They did not postulate that all-round improvements in intelligence scores would come about as a result of listening to Mozart. Two things can be concluded. First, when research is compelling and accessible to the wider media, its message can be corrupted. Second, scientists are reluctant to generalize, so when quality findings emerge they are always tied tightly to the particular circumstances. Engagement with music may lead to some specific improvements in cognitive performance. For example, some musicians, as a result of their training would appear to have a larger left cranial temporal region. This may help with some aspects of verbal memory. This does not make them 'more intelligent'.

'Adults with music training in their childhood demonstrate better verbal memory,' says Dr Agnes Chan of the Chinese University of Hong Kong, who conducted research with 60 female college students, 30 of whom had at least six years training, with one Western musical instrument (such as the violin and the piano) before the age of 12.[62] The other 30 had received no music training. The students were read some words and asked to remember these words – a very common clinical test for memory. Dr Chan describes the outcomes, 'We found that people who have had music training can remember about 17 per cent more information than those who have not had any music training.'

It is believed that this extra ability to remember spoken words is based in a specific part of the brain that is enlarged in musicians. The research, published in the journal *Nature*, is explained by Dr Chan. 'Musicians have asymmetrical left cranial temporal regions of the brain. That is, that part of the brain is relatively larger in musicians than in non-musicians. Some data has suggested that that part of the brain is involved in processing heard information. If that part of the brain is relatively larger, it may be better developed and so this explains very nicely our results.'

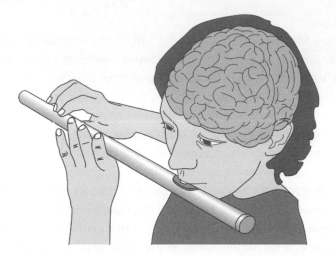

5.4   While playing an instrument such as the flute, the motor and supplementary motor cortex on the left and right is active. The cerebellum is engaged in eye tracking and anticipating movement. The auditory cortex is listening to the sounds played. The frontal cortex is engaged in planning for the combination of physical moves needed to create the desired pattern of sounds.

The brains of trained musicians do, in fact, differ from those of the rest of us. The corpus callosum is larger and so too is the primary motor cortex and the cerebellum. Perhaps this is because of the structured and distributed practice required to be accomplished in any musical instrument combined with the need for smooth and controlled voluntary cross-lateral movement. In other words, you have to use left and right hands simultaneously while thinking about what you are about to do and co-ordinating it with symbols written in front of your eyes. No mean feat! The part of the brain that processes sound (the auditory cortex) in highly skilled musicians is enlarged by about 25 per cent compared with control subjects who have never played an instrument. Enlargement was correlated with the age at which musicians began to practise, suggesting that the reorganization of the auditory cortex is use-dependent.[63]

By practising an instrument you alter the structure of your brain. Non-piano playing adults learned a five-finger exercise on the piano for two hours a day over the course of five days. The area of the brain responsible for finger movements enlarged and become more active in these subjects compared with control subjects who had not learned the piano exercise. This demonstrates that in just five days the adult brain can adapt according to how it is used.[64]

Do you consider yourself to be musical? At what point in your life would you have enough evidence to know? How would it be if we were all musical? Auditions for my Sunday school choir took place in formidable circumstances. The supervisor would line us all up and then listen to us one at a time as we sang. As we were only ten years old at the time, it was highly stressful – especially as one or two of us were encouraged to mime rather than actually sing when the choir eventually performed. A common belief about music is that only a few of us are 'musical', mainly musicians, and that being musical is a 'gift'. The brain research suggests otherwise! Most of our capabilities are not even known to us. They occur in the brain at an unconscious level, so although someone like me will indulge the Sunday school teacher and believe that I have no musical ability, I can never be certain – and isn't that a great thing?

When Stefan Koelsch and his research team from Leipzig analysed brain activation, they found a definite pattern of recognition. Adults who had no musical education and who had never attempted to play a musical instrument were given a series of chords that infrequently contained a chord that did not fit the key implied by the chord sequence. They did not know about chords or key structures and they had no formal musical education and scant musical knowledge.

When all the chords belonged to the same key, their brains showed no special response. When one of the chords did not fit the key that was implied and unconsciously abstracted in their brains, it produced a response that was marked. Puzzled by this, the team repeated the experiment again and again and found the pattern was 'this chord doesn't fit the key'. The brain response occurred although the subjects had no musical training, nor did they know about keys, nor did they know about the belongingness of chords to keys. Their conclusion was that the brain itself seems to make musical sense out of sounds automatically, without prompting and at a level out of conscious awareness.[65] We are all musical!

Kodaly music training uses folk songs and emphasizes melodic and rhythmic elements. In 1975 a year-long study on music and reading was begun with a control group who received extensive music instruction: 40 minutes per day, 5 days a week, for 7 months. A control group of similar age, IQ and socio-economic status had no music training whatsoever. The children were tested on reading ability at the start of the school year and then tested again at the end of the year. After training, the music group exhibited significantly higher reading scores than did the control group, scoring in the 88th percentile vs. the 72nd percentile. The effects also lasted. The music group remained better readers.

Reading is in part about phonological awareness. After a child recognizes the visual symbol, there is a need to relate this symbol to a sound and then get good enough so that the process is automatic. Researchers believe that musical understanding improves recognition of sound changes – the phonemic stage of reading. A recent study by Lamb and Gregory determined the relationship between musical sound discrimination and reading ability in Year 1 children. After a range of different sounding out and sound recognition tests, they found a high degree of correlation between how well children could read both standard and phonic material and how well they could discriminate pitch. Timbre awareness was not related to reading, showing the specificity of the findings. Recognizing change of pitch in the sounds that make up words is thought to be the most important factor in conveying word information. Music training and listening to music develops pitch discrimination.[66]

Doing 'Good Looking'

Does an artist use the same areas of the brain when looking at a Jackson Pollock as I do? I am without any sort of artistic training and no more than an average painter. Some recent research does suggest that the brains of artists work differently to those of other people. Researchers scanned the brain of one of Britain's leading painters, Humphrey Ocean. They asked Mr Ocean to sketch while inside a brain scanner and compared the results with scans of non-artists doing the same thing. The scans revealed the regions of the brain that were most active during the creative process. They found that non-artists tended to use the rear of the brain more. This region is associated with taking in and processing visual information. But Mr Ocean used the frontal cortex of the brain more, the region associated with complex thinking and emotions.

When we look at a picture or an object are we able to be aware of other visual data at the same time? If I am a learner in a classroom, when I watch the teacher can I be seeing something else in my mind's eye at exactly the same time? Or do I have to switch from one set of visual stimuli to another? Is my visual thinking analogue or digital?

Our brain has limited visual processing capacity and yet multiple representations of objects in our visual field are constantly competing with each other. Some researchers have shown that visual clutter actually suppresses the brain's responsiveness. The theory is that by focusing its attention on just one stimulus, the brain cancels out the suppressive influence of nearby stimuli. In this way, it enhances information processing of the desired stimulus.[67] This conflicts with educators who want to create surroundings and texts that are visually rich and often complex.

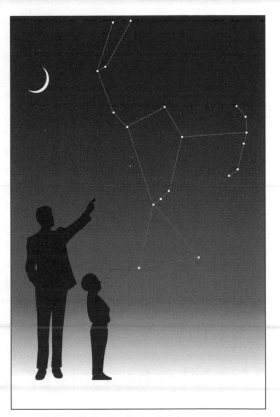

5.5   While visual stimuli is immensely attractive to the brain's specialized centres for recall, it needs to be an active rather than a passive feature of a learning environment.

Subjects in an MRI scanner focused both their eyes and their attention on the lower left corner of a computer screen, while colourfully patterned square-shaped images flashed in the upper right quadrant. The images appeared under two conditions: one at a time, or four simultaneously. As expected, when presented simultaneously, the stimuli evoked weaker responses in the brain than when presented sequentially. This confirmed that multiple stimuli do, in fact, suppress each other. The amount of this mutual suppression progressively increased along a circuit that processes object vision, which runs forwards and downwards from the back of the brain. Neurons at the beginning of this circuit 'see' only a very small portion of the visual field, while neurons near the end respond to almost all of what the eyes see. So neurons at the beginning of the circuit simply could not view the multiple stimuli and were thus spared the suppressive effects. Spacing the images farther apart also decreased suppressive interactions.

Spatially directed attention enhances the brain's visual processing ability by quenching suppression caused by nearby stimuli. What is the significance for educators? Assuming that learners will necessarily assimilate information presented at the periphery of vision is unwise. A visual such as a learning poster needs to have attention directed to it to activate learning. A good visual in a book needs to have attention directed to it for it to best aid recall. It makes a lot of sense to have visual stimulus material that is interactive and requires directed attention. Also, some neurons in object vision see the Big Picture, others are designed to focus on detail. Some learners may be content with digital and small chunk learning but others will need analogue and Big Picture learning. We may have to educate looking: 'looking for learning lessons' with an educator who shows the class how to access and retain visual information, how to take notes visually and spatially, how to revise for an exam using visual tools such as memory maps and learning posters.

Mental rehearsals of success

I was watching the final of the women's high jump at the World Athletics Championships in Edmonton, Canada. At least I was watching it live on television. I saw a pattern of behaviours reminiscent of one of the polar bears that for many years had been a feature at Bristol Zoo. An 'unnatural' pacing up and down, backwards and forwards, again and again: in the case of the bear, all day long; in the case of the athletes, before their turn to jump. What for the bear may have been a release from anxiety and boredom, was, in fact, more purposeful for the athletes.

As I watched I noticed they were mentally rehearsing their stride pattern and their attack on the bar in front of them. One athlete in particular, a South African, fixated her gaze on her imagined stride pattern and with her right hand simulated the movement she wanted her body to take as it successfully cleared the bar. With her head cocked to one side her eyes 'bounced' the stride around the front of the bar – one, two, three, four, five – then spring, hand curving round as she manoeuvred her body over the bar: pause, then again, same routine.

What was the point? In my day the PE teacher encouraged you to take a flyer straight at it, execute a scissors kick, then onto your rear into 15cms of builders' sand – and various other less savoury stuff – and you then spent the next five minutes trying to remove the sand from your underpants. A sports psychologist would say that the body follows the mind. A neuroscientist would say that mental rehearsal is closely related to better motor performance. Experimental psychology has shown us the value of mental rehearsal in advance of performance. It can advantageously affect muscle strength, physical movement, reaction times, speed and timing. Extended rehearsal of tasks in one's head leads to physiological changes such as recovery times, heart and respiration rates. In 1994 research showed that 'motor imagery is closely related to motor preparation'. In other words, becoming ready to ski the downhill course by mentally representing it in sequence engages many of the same structures in the brain as actually ski-ing the course. Many of the same areas of the brain, particularly in the motor cortex, are involved.[68] When scientists have conducted similar experiments involving imagining grasping 3D objects or simulating the movement of a joystick, similar effects have been found.

In November 2001 Guang Yue, an exercise physiologist at the Cleveland Clinic Foundation in Ohio, published findings suggesting that you could strengthen muscles just by imagining yourself exercising. This 'Homer Simpson' approach to exercise will have an appeal to many. It also offers real benefits to those recovering from an injury or a stroke and who might be too weak to go straight back to physical activity. Guang Yue and his team asked ten volunteers to imagine flexing their biceps as hard as they could for as long as they could five times a week. Their brain activity was recorded and so was electrical activity at the motor neurons of the arm muscles. The training lasted three months. After the first two weeks the participants showed an amazing 13.5 per cent increase in upper arm strength and they maintained this until the training stopped. Interviewed about a paper in *Experimental Physiology*, Guang Yue explained that 'muscles move in response to impulses from nearby motor neurons and the firing of these motor neurons depends on the strength of electrical impulses sent by the brain. If this is the case then you can increase muscle strength solely by sending a larger signal to motor neurons from the brain.'[69]

Practice in the skill of mental rehearsal of successful learning behaviours has to be a very powerful endowment to give to any learner. What do your children think of when they hear the word 'test'? Do they rehearse patterns of success or is there a tendency towards mental representations of failure? Here is an area where a direct intervention can be made. Encourage them to capture the 'look' of moments of success and then to rehearse that look again and again. Have them practise successful exam technique in their head. Mentally rehearse coming into the exam room well prepared and relaxed. Feeling confident, sitting down, looking around and relaxing in the familiar surroundings, laying out equipment, opening the exam question paper, reading all the questions, deciding on which to answer and in which order, allocate time by marks, begin each answer with a quick visual plan. All of this can be rehearsed in the head so that it is there in moments of high anxiety.

Chapter 6

Wired to misfire:
learning from dysfunction

This chapter contains the following sections:

不 **How the brain recovers**
How the brain reorganizes itself to compensate for localized damage. Adaptability and plasticity.

不 **Addiction and the brain**
An explanation of addictive behaviours. The concept of 'disinhibition of desire' and the role of the nucleus accumbens. Addiction to nicotine.

不 **Attention–Deficit Hyperactivity Disorder**
Making sense of a confused picture. How deficiencies in attention impact on short- and long-term memory. Some possible strategies for helping children with ADHD.

不 **The roots of aggression**
Case studies showing links between aggressive behaviour and damage to the pre-frontal lobes.

不 **Reading problems**
Some neurological explanations of reading difficulties.

不 **Movement problems**
Poor motor control contributes to learning difficulties. Physical movement can be harnessed to help children learn.

... and will answer the following questions:

- How does a brain cope with trauma? Is full recovery ever possible?

- What happens in the brain when you become addicted? Can you become addicted to non-chemical experiences, such as gambling? What about shopping?

- Is ADHD real?

- Is there something about the brain of an aggressive person that marks it as different?

- Can you explain the major causes of reading problems in children?

- Why will the children in my class not sit still?

Introduction

The case of Martha Curtis, a young musician who suffered epileptic seizures, showed us what happens in the brain during a seizure. During an MRI scan conducted by neurologist Hans Luders, the seizure, as described by John Ratey, 'began as a local electrical disturbance in the right temporal lobe, then spread, eventually taking over her entire brain in a global thunderstorm'.[70] Surgery was required as the seizures had become so severe and so frequent that the drugs prescribed were no longer effective. The area for surgery was to be the right temporal lobe: the area most important in remembering music.

As Ratey describes it, as soon as Martha got out of intensive care, she picked up her violin and tried to play a very difficult Bach piece. She played it 'beautifully'. Sadly the surgeons had not been aggressive enough. The seizures returned. She underwent a second operation and then a third. By the end of the third operation, the neurosurgeons estimated they had removed 20 per cent of the right temporal lobe.

Could she play? She could, and as well as ever. The surgeons concluded that, as a result of measles at age three years, her brain had suffered slight damage and had adapted. For her to become such an accomplished instrumentalist, the centres that would normally be highly active in musical memory had been re-wired and, of necessity, other sites within the brain had adapted to the complex needs. Martha is still an accomplished soloist and a living testimony to the plasticity of the human brain.

How the brain recovers

When scientists talk of the human brain they use adjectives like integrated, complex, adaptive, parallel, holistic and plastic. In a brief study of the indexes of five general books about the workings of the human brain, the word 'plastic' appeared more than any other. What is the significance of this word?

Plasticity is the idea that the brain can reorganize itself to compensate for localized damage. The younger the individual, the more adaptable the brain. The more bilateral the brain, the more it can cope with trauma. Infants with the left hemisphere completely removed before reaching six months old are by age four indistinguishable in language function.[71] Being 'plastic' also means that when a function is lost or inhibited in some way, other parts of the brain can take over that function. Knowing about this helps us understand more about learning difficulties.

Another word often used in relation to studies of the brain is homeostasis. The brain receives information from the external world through the senses and from the internal world through the workings of the body. The brain tries to achieve a constant state and adjusts so there is constancy. This is called homeostasis. The idea that we self-regulate and adjust to what is the norm is important in looking at behaviours and, in particular, 'addictive' behaviours.

Addiction and the brain

Research into addiction is a major, perhaps the major, neurological research industry. There is, quite rightly, great professional caution about premature theorizing. Governments, pharmaceutical companies, alcohol and tobacco manufacturers, customs and excise, sweet and toy manufacturers would all love a silver bullet theory of addiction. There is not one. What we can say is that addictive behaviours are a complex coming together of inherited and learned variables. There are sensitive windows for introducing chemicals to the brain, with consequences for the brain's reward system that can lead to what is described as a 'disinhibition of desire'. Pile on top of this all the socio-economic and family variables, moral opprobrium, the law, what are deemed antisocial behaviours and organized, and even dis-organized, crime and you can see that it is the neurologists who offer most hope of a 'clean' explanation. They have focused this task on the nucleus accumbens.

The nucleus accumbens is a cluster of cells that is highly active in motivation and reward. Located in the forebrain it has direct links to the limbic system. It has a high 'saturation' in neurotransmitters associated with pleasure such as dopamine. Drugs act directly on the nucleus accumbens. These include highly addictive drugs such as cocaine, prescription drugs such as those used to treat ADHD such as Ritalin, everyday drugs such as chocolate, coffee and tea, and occasional drugs such as running, bungee jumping and completing *The Times* crossword. Damage the functioning of the nucleus accumbens and you get a failure of disinhibition. If, for whatever reason, you have an imbalance of chemicals in your nucleus accumbens, homeostasis prompts you to restore the balance. Seeking pleasure or reward, often through novelty, becomes part of your homeostatic response. At this level it is not a conscious choice.

When scientists have been researching the addictive effects of nicotine, they have found that in the West, the vast majority of smokers start during their teenage years. They found that girls were the most vulnerable to addiction and to brain 'damage' and that it can lead to depression. Some studies suggest that starting to smoke early in life can increase the chances of suffering depression in adulthood.

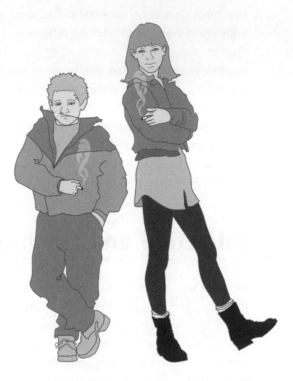

6.1 Addictive behaviours are a complex coming together of inherited and learned variables, with sensitive windows for the reward system. Add to this societal factors and 'inhibition of desire' is a difficult pattern of behaviour to develop. A key role for parents and educators is to foster the ability to manage impulsivity and disinhibition.

Research at Duke University[72] showed that the adolescent brain responds more intensely to nicotine than the adult brain. Working with laboratory rats, the team injected the rats with nicotine every day for more than two weeks to simulate a typical smoker's intake. In every rat the number of chemical receptors dedicated to nicotine increased. This is one way of measuring addiction. In adolescent rats the increase in the number of nicotine receptors was double that of the adult rats.

A follow-up study showed that adolescent exposure to nicotine contributed to subsequent and permanent behavioural problems – especially for females. After two weeks of nicotine, adult female rats that had been injected with the nicotine were more sluggish, less interested in their environment and less interested in looking after their young than adult rats that had no exposure to nicotine.

Possible explanations are that the nicotine had acted as a suppressant and reduced the amounts of dopamine and norepinephrine produced. These chemicals are lower in humans who are suffering from depression. Or, that nicotine retards cell division in the hippocampus, an area of the brain contributing to visual and spatial memory and an area that continues growing into adulthood in females but not in males.

The public face of addiction is that it is all bound up with self-interest, pleasure seeking and reward. Might children who misbehave be addicted to their misbehaviour? Attention-Deficit Hyperactivity Disorder arouses considerable debate among scientists, clinicians and educators alike. The positions taken vary from moral outrage and outright denial through to precise clinical diagnosis. Is there such a thing as ADHD? Are there links with what we know about addictive behaviour?

Attention–Deficit Hyperactivity Disorder

The USA writes 95 per cent of the world's prescriptions for Ritalin, a drug that elevates dopamine levels. Over 3 million children between the ages of 5 and 16 in the USA are deemed to suffer from the disorder. The behaviour patterns that typify ADHD usually arise between the ages of three and five. Even so, the age of onset can vary widely: some children do not develop symptoms until late childhood or even early adolescence.

Boys are at least three times as likely as girls to develop the disorder; indeed, some studies have found that boys with ADHD outnumber girls with the condition by nine to one, possibly because boys are genetically more prone to disorders of the nervous system. Many studies estimate that between 2 and 9.5 per cent of all school-age children worldwide have ADHD.[73]

Opinion varies as to what constitutes ADHD and how, if at all, it should be treated. Many experts are of the view that it is a recognizable neurological condition, that it has been around for longer than its label suggests and that it is treatable through both chemical and non-chemical interventions. Others argue that it is a consequence of poor parenting, inappropriate diet and a culture that promises immediacy of gratification.

In making sense of a confused picture, there seems agreement between those in the neurological camp that it is a deficiency affecting all or some of the components of our attention and reward systems and our memory. In this respect there are many parallels with work done on addiction.

The human attention system comprises four components: arousal, motor orientation, novelty detection and reward, and executive organization. Deficiencies in attention impact on both short- and long-term memory.

A school of thought takes the view that ADHD has its basis in deficiencies in the motivation systems around pleasure and pain and that it is better understood as 'a reward deficiency syndrome': a form of addiction to thrill seeking. The sufferers become besotted with novelty, not because of some moral weakness, but because of an imbalance of chemicals associated with reward – dopamine, serotonin and endorphins – in their brains. Like alcoholics who feel they must drink, ADHD individuals 'seek the intensity of the present because their attention and reward systems are fuelled by the pursuit of immediate pleasures'.[74] High novelty activities provide a temporary surge of dopamine into the brain.

Other researchers have found that children with ADHD are less capable of preparing motor responses in anticipation of events and are insensitive to feedback about errors made in those responses. For example, in a commonly used test of reaction time, children with ADHD are less able than other children to ready themselves to press one of several keys when they see a warning light. They also do not slow down after making mistakes in such tests in order to improve their accuracy.

Some very experienced researchers, including Russell Barkley, Director of Psychology and Professor of Psychiatry and Neurology at the University of Massachusetts Medical Centre, are even more specific.[75] Barkley argues that ADHD arises as 'a developmental failure in the brain circuitry that underlies inhibition and self-control'. He believes that 'loss of self-control in turn impairs other important brain functions crucial for maintaining attention, including the ability to defer immediate rewards for later, greater gain'.

Barkley believes that this 'abstinence aversion' is largely a consequence of an inherited genetic disorder. Areas of the brain that scientists have discovered are significantly smaller in children with ADHD are those that regulate attention. In a 1996 study, F. Xavier Castellanos, Judith L. Rapoport and their colleagues at the National Institute of Mental Health found that the right pre-frontal cortex and two basal ganglia called the caudate nucleus and the globus pallidus are significantly smaller than normal in children with ADHD.[76] The right pre-frontal cortex is involved in 'editing' one's behaviour, resisting distractions and developing an awareness of self and time. The caudate nucleus and the globus pallidus help to switch off automatic responses to allow more careful deliberation by the cortex and to co-ordinate neurological input among various regions of the cortex.

There is a growing body of evidence that ADHD is not caused by chemicals in the diet, poor parenting or electronic games but by genes. Research done by the University of Oslo and the University of Southampton with 526 identical twins, who inherit exactly the same genes, and 389 fraternal twins, who are no more alike genetically than siblings born years apart, found that ADHD has a heritability approaching 80 per cent.[77] A high percentage of the differences in attention, hyperactivity and impulsivity between people with ADHD and those without the disorder can be explained by the genes they inherit.

Furthermore US statistics show that the siblings of children with ADHD are between five and seven times more likely to develop the syndrome than children from unaffected families. And the children of a parent who has ADHD have up to a 50 per cent chance of experiencing the same difficulties.

There are non-genetic factors that contribute to ADHD. These include premature birth, maternal alcohol and tobacco use, exposure to high levels of lead in early childhood and brain injuries – especially those that involve the pre-frontal cortex. But, even together, these factors can account for only between 20 and 30 per cent of ADHD cases among boys; among girls, they account for an even smaller percentage.

When scientists compare the symptoms of ADHD with those of frontal lobe damage there is a remarkable consistency.

Both ADHD and frontal lobe damage patients are easily distracted, highly erratic in attention, have poor social inhibition, often intrude and self-talk inappropriately.

The frontal lobes are highly involved in social inhibition. The frontal lobes are not fully developed until early adulthood. Some scientists think that the frontal lobes mature more slowly in some than in others. As a general principle, activation levels in the brain go down as you become more expert.

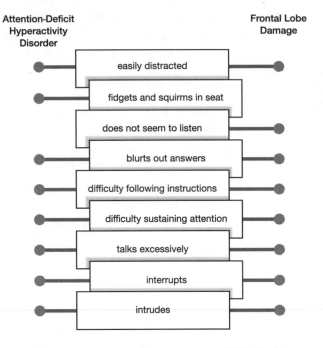

6.2   A comparison of the symptoms of ADHD with those of frontal lobe damage.

Frontal lobe function is maintained by dopamine. Scientists such as Barkley are of the opinion that genes responsible for the secretion of dopamine in the brain are defective and that this contributes to these behaviours. Dopamine is secreted by neurons in specific parts of the brain to inhibit or modulate the activity of other neurons, particularly those involved in emotion and movement. Some impressive studies specifically implicate genes that encode, or serve as the blueprint for, dopamine receptors and transporters; these genes are very active in the pre-frontal cortex and basal ganglia. These are areas of the brain that are directly involved in managing impulsive response, resisting distractions and goal-setting.

Barkley has a very interesting and useful hypothesis as to what happens next. He identifies the internalization of executive functions of self-control as something that does not fully develop in children with ADHD. He says that this is largely caused by genetic mutations that affect those parts of the brain involved in self-control.

To exercise this 'self-control' children need:

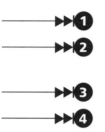

1. their working memory to be functional.

2. to be able to 'talk themselves' through things in their heads.

3. to control emotions, motivation and mood.

4. to learn from observed experience.

To develop 'self-control' with children who exhibit ADHD, parents and teachers should be aware of what leads to their behaviours.

1 Memory
When children are unable to direct their attention to an activity for any length of time, we have problems with short-term memory. Children need to be able to hold information in their heads while working on a task, particularly when the original stimulus has gone. If children cannot do this, then information will not be transferred to long-term memory. Life for such children will be constantly in the present. Remembering is crucial for learning chains of consequence, for setting goals for the future, for learning through reflection and for anticipating the future. Remembering is also important for

imitation and learning through observation and rehearsal. All these functions are drastically limited in children with ADHD.

2 Self-talk

A normal part of growing up is being able to talk yourself through something in your head. When children are young this 'executive function' is performed aloud. Children talk themselves through a task aloud. This is good for learning and it is natural. It is also more prevalent in girls than in boys. As children grow up, the thoughts are internalized and become part of their thinking skills. Children with ADHD lack the restraint to internalize their thinking and continue to externalize their thoughts. Tourette's syndrome is an exaggerated version of this problem. Before the age of 6, most children talk aloud to themselves, reminding themselves how to perform a particular task or trying to cope with a problem. It evolves into private muttering, and by the age of ten is no longer heard.[78] Researchers at Illinois State University reported in 1991 that the internalization of self-directed speech is delayed in boys with ADHD.

3 Managing impulsivity

Children need to learn to adjust their behaviour according to the circumstances. This adaptability needs to be learned and practised. In order to learn and practise it, children must be able to regulate their own emotional responses. Managing the moment of impulse is, for some, an intelligent behaviour of the highest order. Accident victims with frontal lobe damage frequently have problems doing this. In many cases, they are unable to discern the motivation of others. They often lock into a cycle of impulsivity, recklessness and aggression. In order to complete a learning task, a child may have to manage or delay an emotional response to a potential distraction. This requires strong internal resources. A child with ADHD does not yet have such internal resources.

4 Safe rehearsal

Children with ADHD have to work very hard to learn from others. They need to observe the behaviours of those around and then break those behaviours down into 'rules'. These 'rules' then need to be reconstituted into actions that are new for the ADHD child. This is complex, demanding and requires time. To be able to do this is what motivation and goal-setting is all about. Children work towards their goal without having to learn all the steps by rote. It becomes a learned response through rehearsal. To rehearse it safely, it needs to be done privately and again and again. As you practise it becomes a reflexive response. You always do it that way. As children get older, and by means of safe rehearsal, they ought to become better at chaining together behaviours across longer and longer intervals to secure a goal. Initial studies suggest that children with ADHD are less capable of safe rehearsal and reconstitution than are other children.

Children with ADHD are often prescribed drugs such as Ritalin. Prescriptions in the UK have gone up by more than 45 times in the six-year period from 2,000 in 1991 to 92,000 in 1997. In the USA, 3 per cent of children with ADHD are given the drug. These psychostimulants act by inhibiting the dopamine transporter, increasing the time that dopamine has to bind to its receptors on other neurons. This boosts the child's capacity to regulate impulsive response, which, in turn, helps them resist distractions, hold information longer in short-term memory and rehearse goal-setting. Drugs such as Ritalin have been found to improve the behaviour of between 70 and 90 per cent of children with ADHD older than five years. As a result of better self-control, these children attract less censure from adults and peers and therefore begin to be liked more.

Surely our first strategy as parents or as teachers is to create structure in the lives of children, who, through no fault of their own, have poor experience of coping with structure? This could be done by:

 defining the benefits of completing a task rather than the task's features.

 breaking the task down into achievable chunks.

practising self-talk, aloud at first then quieter and quieter.

lots of rehearsals to embed information into short-term memory.

practising time lines.

 practising goal-setting throughout and insist that the child articulates the goal to you.

 gradually extending the goals.

praising for very specific, perhaps small, improvements.

The roots of aggression

It is naïve to assume that all aggressive behaviour can be traced to an impairment in functioning somewhere within the brain. The causes of aggressive behaviour in humans are many and varied and this needs to be acknowledged. However, systems within the brain do operate with greater or lesser effect to manage impulsivity and to allow thinking space for more considered response.

Aggressive people often have underactive frontal lobes, the areas of the brain that restrain impulsive action and that inform reasoned thought. Damage to these frontal lobes can lead to irresponsible behaviour. Inability to manage impulse can lead to a cycle of impulsivity, recklessness and aggression. Some very recent research on damage to the part of the brain that learns moral and social rules – the pre-frontal cortex – could cause children to grow up into irresponsible adults and even exhibit criminal behaviour.

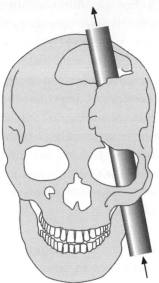

6.3 Phineas Gage has become a *cause célèbre* in neuroscience. His skull is preserved in the Smithsonian Museum and clearly shows the serious damage caused by the tamping rod.

Phineas Gage was a railway worker who, in 1848, suffered terrible but not fatal injuries when a tamping rod with which he was tamping down some dynamite caused an explosion. This metal rod was driven with such brutal force that it went clean through his pre-frontal cortex. Before the accident he had been industrious, dependable and well liked, but afterwards he became a drifter who was profane, unreliable, impulsive and inconsiderate to his family. His intellectual capacities nevertheless remained intact. He could articulate answers to complex questions, he could reason and he understood cause and effect. But after his accident his moral behaviour was distressing to family and friends.

The man had changed beyond recognition. He survived for many years through exhibiting himself, his wound and the tamping rod in circuses throughout America. Eventually he died alone, penniless, an alcoholic.

In more recent times, research published in *Nature Neuroscience* by neuroscientists from the University of Iowa focused on the case studies of two individuals who had suffered damage to the pre-frontal cortex as babies.[79] One was a girl aged 20, who had been knocked down by a car at 15 months. The other was a man aged 23, who had undergone brain surgery at three months. In each case the children made full recoveries and were able to enjoy an upbringing that was advantaged. They were nurtured in middle-class families with educated parents. However, on reaching puberty, their behaviour began to change. Whereas before they had been dutiful, considerate of others and seemingly content, now they lied, behaved selfishly, were lazy and disruptive. In school they started fights and stole money. They also became sexually reckless, becoming parents of children that they then neglected. In both cases, the brain's normal cognitive functions, such as reading and writing, were unaffected. What was affected was an ability to realize the social consequences of misbehaviour and to carry out moral reasoning.

One of the most interesting findings was a difference between those people brain injured as children and those damaged as adults. The adult patients understood moral and social rules but appeared unable to apply them to their own lives. Those damaged at an early age seemed unable to learn the rules in the first place, having as adults the moral reasoning skills of ten year olds. They were also more likely to exhibit psychopathic behaviour such as stealing and being violent.

Another intriguing finding is that patients with these problems do not learn lessons from being punished after misbehaving. This could call into question the effectiveness of criminal penalties when applied to this group. Two is a very small sample but it is hard to find documented cases where brain damage has such restricted effects.

Very low or very high levels of serotonin in the brain can also contribute to aggression. Without modifiers to dampen down the bonfires of impulsive response we become prone to impulsivity, recklessness and aggression.

Serotonin imbalance can be treated with SSRIs (selective serotonin reuptake inhibitors) such as Prozac. High levels of testosterone can also lead to aggression. A deadly combination is when there are unusually low levels of serotonin alongside high levels of testosterone. Dion Sanders is a young man currently serving a life sentence without parole in a US prison in Ohio for the murder of his grandparents. His crime was particularly violent, but he claimed not to have knowledge of just how violent. He agreed to allow a spinal tap to look at the prevalence of neurotransmitters in his system. Scientists discovered this rare combination of low levels of serotonin alongside high levels of testosterone in Sanders. His death sentence was commuted to life.

Reading problems

In the UK about 5 per cent of children have difficulty learning to speak and about 20 per cent of children have difficulty learning to read. Both require acquisition of phonological skills that depend on sensitive auditory perception of frequency and amplitude changes in speech sounds. Girls and boys appear to differ in the way language is acquired and developed. Girls usually say their first words and learn to speak in sentences earlier than boys. Some studies have found that women speak in longer, more complex sentences than men. Also, boys outnumber girls in remedial reading classes. Stuttering and other speech defects occur more frequently among males.

The brain is not designed to be literate, that is a socially constructed phenomenon, but it is designed for language. Becoming literate does, however, have consequences for the structure of the brain. If I was to give two pieces of advice to a parent, the first would be to monitor your child's health and the second would be to talk to, with and around your child frequently and positively. We used a saying earlier 'you build your house and then you live in it'. This is especially true of the brain and language. If it is possible to re-wire a brain, and I think it is, then the early acquisition of language has to be the most potent force for doing so. Television, video and computers do not make good baby sitters. In less than 2000 years mothers in some Western countries have gone from spending 24 hours in the company of their young children to, in some cases, two or three hours of quality time. That is a lot less language exchange.

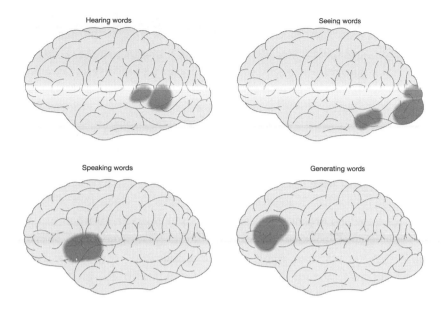

6.4   When scanned using PET, different areas of the brain are activated by a reading task. Activity in the primary auditory cortex and in Wernicke's area is increased when hearing words. Seeing words activates the visual cortex. Speaking words activates the primary motor cortex. Generating words activates Broca's area.

Longitudinal research conducted in Kansas and in Alaska attempted to quantify typical exposure to language. Todd Risley and Betty Hart led a project that compared children from different types of family background.[80] They looked at welfare, blue- and white-collar families and found a startling pattern of difference in exposure to language. By the age of four, children in the welfare families had as many as 13 million fewer words of cumulative language experience compared to their peers in the blue- and white-collar families.

In an experiment conducted in Portugal, literate and illiterate women were compared.[81] The women, who were elderly and from similar social backgrounds, were asked to listen to and repeat simulated words and real words. The brain areas that showed activity were the same in both groups for real words but differed for the artificial words. In the brains of those who were literate the artificial words were treated like familiar and real words, whereas in those who had no literacy the brain areas activated were different and to do with memory retrieval. At a level beyond everyday recognition, the brain was showing recognition patterns by the areas activated. With no recognition, lots of resources were directed towards finding and securing a match from memory. Become literate and you use your brain more efficiently. The corpus callosum, a structure within the brain that conduits signals across the two hemispheres of the cortex, tends to be thinner and has less neural density in illiterates.

Dyslexia is a real phenomenon. In recent years research has shown that it is a developmental disorder with its origin in genetic inheritance. It is also culturally shaped insofar as different languages place different demands on brain function. What is interesting about this is the idea that different cultures shape and organize different brains and especially so when you are an active user of language within that culture. There is no single physical cause that has yet been recognized as the 'signature' of dyslexia, but a pattern of brain abnormalities that come together in the processing of language has been observed by a number of scientists. One of the features that distinguishes the brains of dyslexics is the degree to which a language area in the brain is asymmetric. During reading tasks, an area of the brain in the left temporal lobe that would normally show high levels of activity in organizing sounds into words and also in retrieving those words from memory is less active in dyslexics generally.

The English language has a great number of irregularities in grammatical construction and in the rules of spelling. To become a skilled reader in English requires different patterns of brain activation than becoming a skilled reader in Italian. English dyslexics have a harder time learning to read. Research conducted by Paulesu showed that both groups used the same structures in the left hemisphere.[82] Italian readers used more of the superior temporal gyrus, which is involved in translating sounds into letters. English readers used more of the inferior basal temporal areas and anterior regions of the frontal gyrus, which are areas involved in interpreting word meaning. Why should there be any difference? What significance might there be?

Because English has many spelling irregularities and more variations in the grammatical rules than Italian, it requires more effort in de-coding meaning and less in linking sounds to letters than Italian. Although, in the experiment reported, no irregular words were presented, the English readers engaged more areas associated with word identity rather than sound-letter de-coding.

A knowledge of irregular words – 'we went' instead of 'we goed' – becomes necessary before they can be successfully pronounced. Differences in brain structures are subtle, but are a reflection of the uses to which they are put. Does this mean that teaching Italian and teaching English necessitates different teaching methods?

Most classroom instruction is orally based. If you are equipped with poor mechanisms for recognizing, separating, remembering and replicating sounds, you will struggle in a classroom. Children with poor phonemic awareness will become slow readers. According to Torgesen children in the bottom 20 per cent in phonological awareness at age five are likely to be two and an half years behind in their reading age by the time they are ten years old.[83] The left hemispheres of dyslexics appear to be particularly susceptible to abnormalities such as ectopias. These arise before birth and can be related to autoimmune disorders. For children with this inherited abnormality normal learning of speech sound and sound-to-letter de-coding is very difficult.

Problems can be compounded by poor verbal short-term memory and by poor eye tracking. According to Professor John Stein, Professor of Neurology at Oxford University, 'more than half of dyslexic children may have eye control problems'.[84] Some can be helped with eye patches, or coloured spectacles, or coloured overlays that go on top of the reading material. As I write, state-of-the-art 'eye wobble' diagnosis spectacles are in trial. Adapted from cockpit control systems where pilots direct missiles with their eyes, the kits use tiny video cameras linked to computers and are attached to spectacle frames to assess eye tracking. If a child has 'eye wobble', then he is unlikely to be able to move his eyes steadily along a line of text. Remedial eye exercises can then be prescribed. Early diagnosis is crucial and, according to the British Dyslexia Association, only 11 per cent of schools in the UK

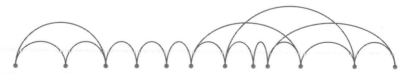

When reading the eyes do not move in a straight flowing line.

6.5 When reading the eyes do not move in a straight flowing line but in a series of small jumps known as saccades. Children with poor eye tracking can be given some help by practising tracking exercises.

routinely screen for dyslexia. Simple tests that already exist can pinpoint youngsters with dyslexia by the time they start school.

Changing the reading scheme does not work. New teaching methods might. Fast ForWord is a computer-based program designed to improve the brain's capacity for identifying, separating, remembering and replicating sounds. Computers are better at doing some things than humans. The computer is used to replicate ideal learning conditions. Starting as early as possible Fast ForWord is an intervention to help dyslexics and those with genuine reading difficulties. The best form of computer-aided learning for a disability, according to those behind Fast ForWord:

- is intensive
- is distributed
- is frequent
- requires a motor response
- reinforces correct responses
- is gradual
- progressively works towards a targeted goal.

The phoneme is the smallest unit of sound related to word meaning that the brain must recognize. If, as a result of an injury or inherited disorder, the child's brain is poorly equipped for discriminating sound changes and the beginnings and endings of sounds, then we have a reading problem stored for the future. The computerized programs alter the pattern of word sounds to exaggerate beginnings and endings and stretch out the sounds in between. The child sits with headphones in front of a screen and completes sound exercises, phoneme exercises and word exercises. 'Old McDonald's Flying Farm' is a sound exercise where children click the mouse when they notice a different phoneme hidden among many acoustically modified to sound similar. 'Phonic Match' requires them to distinguish between, and remember, similar real and imaginary words. 'Block Commander' builds listening and attention skills by asking them to take part in a game where there are carefully chosen and increasingly challenging acoustically controlled commands.

Another very different form of intervention is the use of carefully constructed physical exercises to improve eye tracking. The cerebellum in the back of the brain contributes to balance, eye tracking and anticipatory movement. Exercises such as balancing on a wobble board, using hula hoops, cross crawling, lying on your tummy on top of a large inflatable ball and rocking back and forth have been shown to have helped the reading, writing and spelling of a control group of 50 children aged 6 to 18.[85] For the group as a whole, reading skills progressed at a rate of 67 per cent compared to a control group. Progress in writing was 32 per cent higher and in spelling 42 per cent.

Movement problems

Dyspraxia is a word with which you are probably not familiar. It is a further 'dys' to add to a growing list of words that describe a specific learning difficulty. The word 'praxis' has its origins in Greek and means 'to do'. Dyspraxia is a difficulty affecting voluntary movement and co-ordination. The term 'Developmental Dyspraxia' describes a wider spectrum of difficulties, including problems of language, perception and thought.

The cerebellum plays a leading role in movement. Learning a motor skill utilizes the cerebellum. As the child practises crawling, the gross motor movements are rehearsed, adjusted, repeated and improved. Adjustments become finer and finer, the movements quicker and more precise. Children who have the slightest damage to the cerebellum do not make this same steady progress. Impairments in the cerebellum can lead to difficulties in co-ordinating movement, catching a ball, tapping out a rhythm, balancing on a beam, skipping and playing a percussion instrument.

In her book *Developmental Dyspraxia*, Madeleine Portwood, a UK-based educational psychologist, suggests that about 6 per cent of all youngsters are dyspraxic and have difficulties that are sufficiently significant to require intervention.[86] In the UK four boys to every girl are diagnosed as dyspraxic. In countries where there is a greater emphasis on physical movement and developing gross motor skills as part of early education, the incidence of dyspraxia is reported at 1 per cent. Portwood is very careful to point out that all children have a different developmental trajectory and that being disorganized, forgetful and clumsy is part of growing up! Accurate diagnosis of a problem is difficult and requires a variety of tests.

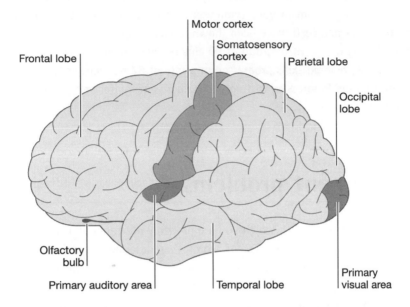

Motor cortex

Somatosensory cortex

Frontal lobe

Parietal lobe

Occipital lobe

Olfactory bulb

Primary auditory area

Temporal lobe

Primary visual area

6.6 The motor control strip and the cerebellum control voluntary movement. Early introduction to co-ordinated motor movements that are deliberate, smooth and controlled contributes to improvements in all-round cognitive functioning.

Among the observable behaviours of youngsters around school age are those to do with social skills, gross and fine motor skills, reasoning ability and language skills. A child who is dyspraxic may be naïve about social codes and indulge in intentional spoiling, aggressiveness to others, physical roughness and inability to defer gratification. This combination of difficulties allied to physical awkwardness may mean that the child gets excluded from group games and becomes even more isolated. The dyspraxic child is more accident prone than his classmates. When he attempts to throw a ball his other hand makes a similar movement; while sitting at his desk he swings his legs and fidgets. Although he knows how to assemble the jigsaw, he cannot master the delicate sequence of movements to do so. Simple rules of eating are also hard to follow. Portwood says that language delay can usually be traced to 'a motor problem in the way that the lips, tongue and palate co-ordinate to produce the sound'. If you understand the world around you but cannot communicate that understanding to those whom you would have as friends, it can cause emotional problems. Problems with sequencing, concepts of cause and effect, understanding time and following instructions arise as a result of poorer neurological functioning. The brain's internal messaging system is working but more slowly.

When a child 'practises' a complex motor movement such as painting, neural structures associated with seeing, with moving the hands and with remembering the 'look' of the original are involved. With practice, and with fine adjustments to the skill, more and more neurons in nearby structures are recruited to the task. We become more adept.

Motor memory works when the frontal cortex anticipates and plans for the movement and recruits the basal ganglia and the hippocampus for memory of similar movements in the past: it is then that the cerebellum and motor control strip are activated to ensure smooth progression of the movement. Early introduction to co-ordinated motor movements that are deliberate, smooth and controlled enhances all-round cognitive functioning. Again and again, studies into teaching a musical instrument, teaching dance, teaching the movement rules of a sport or teaching choral singing have pointed to improved levels of hemispheric integration. In other words, use it or lose it and start doing so early! This allows the brain to become better at communicating with itself. In the absence of this provision then intervention through physical activity is important. Distributed practice with structured motor movements can help.

Chapter **7**

Wired to retire:
ageing and the brain

This chapter contains the following sections:

⽊ Hardening of the attitudes
How to avoid cognitive loss with ageing. How learning can reduce cell death in the brain by as much as 45 per cent.

⽊ The network's down
A summary of what happens with degenerative conditions such as Alzheimer's disease.

⽊ Stay active
The importance of physical activity to the brain. How stress in old age has a disproportionate impact on intellectual performance. Heart disease.

⽊ Hold on to what you've got
Why procedural learning resists memory loss more than any other type.

⽊ Sagging, wrinkling, shrinking
As we age the brain shrinks, particularly in males. What are the consequences?

... and will answer the following questions:

➤ What is the impact of new learning on the brain of an elderly person?

➤ Is there anything that can be done to delay Alzheimer's disease?

➤ How does stress affect memory in old age?

➤ How is it that an elderly lady who cannot remember her own name can nevertheless remember how to knit?

➤ Why is it that as we age the brain shrinks in males but not in females?

Introduction

Norman Wisdom has huge popularity in Albania. There is something about this small, socially awkward, physically inept underdog that appeals to their population. When the English national soccer team played a World Cup qualifier in the capital Tirane, the ageing actor got the biggest cheer of the night when he came onto the pitch before the game started. Norman Wisdom is now an octagenarian. He was recently knighted for his services to the entertainment industry. When he was interviewed about the honour he said, 'As you get older three things go, the first is your memory and I can't remember the other two.'

Can an understanding of ageing and the brain tell us anything about learning? The answer is 'yes'. A great deal of effort and money goes into research into ageing and the brain worldwide. This is particularly true of illnesses of dementia. Scientists have not produced many careful studies of how environment affects dementia, but those who have offer some insights into learning.

Hardening of the attitudes

Studies into ageing and memory suffer from the cohort problem. The cohort problem in a nutshell is this: the life experience of a group of people who are now in their 70s is radically different from that of a similar sample who are now in their 30s. In order to compare memory it is best to compare Mrs Smith now with Mrs Smith when she was 30. The comparative data that does exist suggests memory in older people seems to be better now than it was in older people 70 years ago.

To stay healthy and live longer, then stay fit and intellectually challenged. 'The only guaranteed antidote to Alzheimer's is to extend the number of years we actively participate in education.' This quote, from an Oxford University neurologist, suggests that the sustained cognitive challenge that some elderly people still put into their lives keeps them healthy.[87] The challenge of learning encourages cell growth and reduces neural atrophy.

Research completed by Dr Matthew During and his team from Thomas Jefferson University in Philadelphia shows that a stimulating environment combined with early and continued learning both protects the brain from disease and increases its ability to re-grow damaged cells. 'We've shown that a learning environment can encourage cell growth and also reduce cell death as well by about 45 per cent,' says Dr During.[88]

During and his colleagues performed experiments in which rats lived for several weeks in either standard housing or 'enrichment housing' – filled with running wheels, tunnels, balls and choices of food. The researchers treated rats with a seizure-inducing neurotoxin. They found that rats housed in the enriched environment were almost completely protected against seizures. The rate of neural atrophy – cell death – in the hippocampal areas of the brains of rats in the standard housing was 45 per cent higher than those in the enriched environments. The hippocampus contributes to learning via long-term memory.

During believes these findings suggest that 'an enriched environment switched on protective genes in the brain'. Through this mechanism, he explained, 'the brain becomes super-resilient, more resistant to ageing and diseases, such as Alzheimer's, Parkinson's, and traumatic brain injury'.

Some people worry that as we age we lose our ability to remember things. Some loss of memory function is natural but not to a significant and noticeable degree before about 70 years of age. Long-term memory seems to suffer little while working memory, the day-to-day momentary things, is much more affected. As we age the weight of the brain decreases. Parts of the hippocampus atrophy as we age but there is no significant global neural decay. Some people believe that this is because the basal forebrain becomes less efficient and so produces less acetylcholine.

As Professor Nick Rawlins of Oxford University puts it, 'all memory capacities are not affected by ageing in the same way'.[89] He points out some of the differences:

- Skill learning can be preserved when explicit learning is going.
- Recognition stays longer than recall.

- You remember the context or the source of the memory – it becomes part of you.

- Implicit memory is spared when explicit is lost.

Stress seems to have a differential effect on older people's memory performance. When pushed hard in simple memory activities, recall drops. When given time and more relaxed circumstances recall is restored.

The network's down

Contrary to popular belief, no more than 10 to 15 per cent of people aged 65 plus suffer from senile dementia. Professor Robert Sapolsky describes the effects of Alzheimer's on memory function like this, 'with Alzheimer's memory is not lost, it takes more effort to get the memory out. We require more and more priming cues and stronger and stronger cueing pulls the memory out'.[90]

There are not enough neurons for each cell to be able to just recognize one stimulus. Cells work in assemblies or what are called 'networks'. Ageing impacts on these networks. Some of the networks are there and some are not. It is like trying to telephone conference on cellular phones when one or two of those phones stray out of signal: messages are incomplete, only partly or poorly sent or received, or missing altogether.

As we age we also lose some function in the frontal lobes – neuron atrophy, reduction in blood flow and glucose metabolism – and become less efficient at remembering the order and timing of events.

Decline in dopamine means that neurons become less efficient at receiving messages. Dopamine is the brain's natural reward system. Its loss might be part of the cause of 'narrowing of horizons' that occurs in old age. Or might 'narrowing of horizons' in old age be the cause of a loss in dopamine?

Harvard Medical School Professor Marilyn Albert says our memory changes as we age.[91] The biggest change is that we can absorb less per hour. If you spread out the learning, giving 20-minute breaks, the ability to retain information is good. Naturally if a person has Alzheimer's, the brain does not normally transfer the learning to long-term memory. One of the keys to the preservation of memory as we age is to enhance blood flow through exercise.

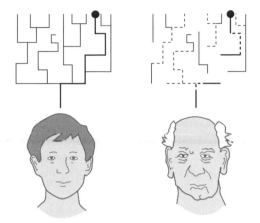

7.1   When the network goes down it is not that the memories are not there, it is just that they require stronger and more varied cueing to assemble their elements together.

Stay active

Inactivity can contribute to, and arise from, depression. This is a vicious cycle that some elderly people find themselves locked into as a result of some profound change in their lives: the death of a partner, the isolation of an old people's home, retirement. There is strong evidence to show that depression can cause shrinkage of the hippocampus in the elderly. The size of the hippocampus averaged 14 per cent smaller in a group of septuagenarians who showed high and rising cortisol levels, compared to a group with moderate and decreasing levels.[92] Cortisol is a stress hormone. Depression generates stress.

They also did worse at remembering a path through a human maze and pictures they had seen 24 hours earlier – two tasks that use the hippocampus.

A third of the 60 volunteers, who were between ages 60 and 85, had chronically high cortisol levels, a problem that seems to be fairly common in older people. Cortisol also interferes with the function of neurotransmitters, the chemicals that brain cells use to communicate with each other. This makes it difficult to think or access long-term memories. That is why some people get befuddled and confused in a severe crisis: their mind goes blank because 'the lines are down'.

Professor Robert Sapolsky's research with animals also showed that an excess of stress-related hormones causes further problems for the elderly.[93] The problems included 'fatigue, thinning muscles, adult-onset diabetes, hypertension, osteoporosis and immune suppression'.

Professor Sapolsky concluded that 'Aged organisms not only have trouble turning off the stress-response after the end of stress, they also secrete more

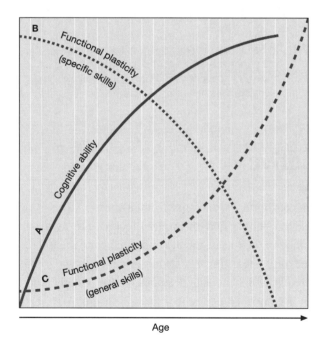

7.2   Line A shows how cognitive ability increases from birth through adulthood and begins to flatten out in old age. Line B shows how functional plasticity for specific skills diminishes from birth through adulthood. Line C shows how functional plasticity for general skills increases from birth through adulthood.

stress-related hormones even in their normal, non-stressed state ... Old individuals of all sorts tend to have the stress-response turned on even when nothing stressful is happening.'

As we age the speed at which we store new information slows. Our capacity to deal with changes in routine suffers and so does our ability to transfer information. Elderly people who have a lifetime of effective learning methods such as categorizing, storing, retrieving and transferring behind them tend to remain better. Their memory is less susceptible to impaired function because it has been used more efficiently over an extended period of time.

It is a good idea as we age to monitor our lifestyle. Smoking combined with obesity will not only cause heart disease but also contribute to a decline in learning performance too.

Professor Merrill Elias of Boston University School of Medicine, who led the research into risk factors and mental prowess, said, 'We want people to function at the highest possible level and for the longest possible time. Individuals are going to have a reduced quality of life if they cannot learn and remember.'[94]

Professor Elias's group tested 1,799 volunteers involved in the Framingham Heart Study, which has tracked the cardiovascular health of a group of residents in a community near Boston for about 50 years. The study showed that the more risk factors for heart disease a person has, the greater the risk of developing memory and learning impairments. The risk factors were smoking, obesity, high blood pressure and diabetes.

After analysing the scores on tests they found that people with one of four risk factors at the time of testing were, on average, 23 per cent more likely to be poor performers than those with no risk factors. With each additional risk factor, the volunteer's risk of decreased mental function increased another 23 per cent. The tests measured learning and memory, attention, concentration and word fluency. Writing in the US journal *Health Psychology*, Professor Elias's team found that in 140 participants studied over 20 years, all showed a decline in mental ability. But they also found that the higher the subject's blood pressure, the faster the decline.

Hold on to what you've got

How is it that a frail old lady suffering from dementia and unable to remember her son's name, the fact that he lives with his new wife 50 miles away and the fact that her partner pre-deceased her four years previously can, nevertheless, crochet and knit? How is it that the memory of names, faces, places, facts and everyday trivia can be so fragile but the memory of rehearsed motor movement seems so stubborn? How can it be that a physical movement or an involuntary gesture can precipitate a chain of associated but since forgotten memories?

Acquiring a physical skill is known as procedural learning and it is different – even dissociated – from acquiring factual knowledge.[95] Recent imaging studies would seem to confirm this. Patients with amnesia are often unable to learn and retain new facts but they can often acquire new physical skills and in many cases will be able to access physical things they could do before their brain damage. Amnesic patients are also able to acquire new skills, and this despite not remembering how or when they were taught the skill. How is such a phenomena to be explained?

It is down to an area of the brain known as the basal ganglia. The basal ganglia is often intact after trauma has damaged other sites within the brain. If so, it remains capable of procedural learning, demonstration of that learning and access to previously rehearsed skills. Patients who have Parkinson's disease and whose basal ganglia is damaged, can remember facts and episodic information but have difficulty learning new skills. This suggests that there is a separate set of systems operating for the memory of procedural skills from that of acquiring and retaining factual knowledge. A 'dissociation' thus exists between declarative and procedural learning.

This leads to a key question for educators. Factual learning and physical learning occurs separately: why? Might there not be efficiencies in combining both modes to access and retain new information? If we learn historical dates through a combination of procedural and declarative memory, would we not multiply up the chances of recalling the dates? Observing effective classroom practice over many years has pointed me to the answer: a resounding yes!

Sagging, wrinkling, shrinking

If you are a mother, did you become forgetful during pregnancy? Cannot remember? You are forgiven, you probably had other things on your mind and, besides, your brain was smaller at the time. Research at the Royal Postgraduate Medical School in London showed that women's brains shrink 3–5 per cent during pregnancy. In tests, more than 70 per cent of women had difficulty learning new information during their ninth month of pregnancy. During pregnancy, performances on spatial and verbal tests were 15–20 per cent lower. Six months later, the brain, and the scores, had returned to normal. However, there was no conclusive evidence that the partner's brain also shrinks during the hours of labour.

Finally, as if there was not enough sagging, wrinkling and shrinking involved with ageing, it appears that the male brain shrinks faster with age than the female brain. Men are more prone to memory loss as they age. Might a shrinking brain contribute to this?

Human brains reach their full size in adolescence and begin shrinking after age 20. As the brain gets smaller, the amount of fluid between the brain and skull increases. Between the ages of 65 and 95, men had a 30 per cent increase in fluid, but women only had a 1 per cent increase. People who have high cholesterol, who have one or more alcoholic drinks a day and who smoke, speed the process. As a general rule, according to the report's author, Dr C. Edward Coffey, a neuropsychiatrist at Henry Ford Behavioural Services in Michigan, the brain shrinks at about 10 per cent every 10 years.[96] The brain shrinkage and fluid increase were mostly seen in the frontal and temporal lobes, which control thinking, planning and memory. Dr Coffey, who used MRI to measure the brains of 330 healthy men and women, also found that women are better at holding on to verbal memories, while men are better at non-verbal skills, like map-reading or putting a puzzle together. He also noted varying rates of shrinkage particularly among those over the age of 60. An explanation is proving elusive.

2

PART TWO

Ready, wire, fire: a model for
the learning brain

Chapter **8**

Physiology:
how do we maintain the brain?

This chapter contains the following sections:

⊼ **The brain marches on its stomach**
How girls' diet can lower their exam performance. Why iron intake is so important. Schools with breakfast clubs. What happens when you bolt your food.

⊼ **The water solution**
Does drinking water help you concentrate? Should water fountains be restored to classrooms? Surprising findings about the temperature of drinking water and exams.

⊼ **Sleep, learning and the brain**
How sleep is vital to learning. What happens to the brain in sleep. Boys in late adolescence and sleep delay syndrome.

⊼ **Movement, play and learning**
Evidence that movement and play alters brain structure advantageously. Why movement is an integral part of the best learning. Schools should argue a stronger case for structured play.

⊼ **You've got to laugh about it**
The link between laughter and learning. The world's funniest joke. The therapeutic value of laughter.

⊼ **Sing when you are winning**
How singing improves your resistance to illness. The feel-good factor behind singing and why doing it together is best.

... and will answer the following questions:

- If I skip breakfast will it impair my thinking?

- Is there any real evidence that drinking water improves children's classroom learning?

- How does sleep improve all-round memory and recall?

- What scientific evidence can I call on to argue the case for structured play in the early years classroom?

- Is there any evidence that laughter helps learning?

- I feel better when I have been singing. Why?

Introduction

In excess of a hundred different neurotransmitter varieties have been identified in the brain, and others are continually being discovered. It seems that each one probably plays some role in shaping behaviours. In general, a neurotransmitter is identified by whether it either excites or inhibits – in various degrees – the nerve impulse in target neurons. The little electrical signals sent by neurons down the axon will arrive at the synapse, or junction, but will not be able to cross the junction until the correct neurotransmitters are in place and ready to connect to receptors.

There is a biochemical mating game that occurs between the neurotransmitters and the receptors in target neurons. The neurotransmitter wants to meet the receptor on the receiving neuron, but there are lots of them. With the right chemical match, the neurotransmitter sticks. This extraordinary mating game of neurotransmitter and receptor influences every aspect of your behaviour. It is all influenced by what you eat.

The brain marches on its stomach

A brain marches on its stomach. Neurotransmitters are made from the amino acids contained in dietary proteins. Proteins are the building blocks of the animal kingdom, and amino acids are the building blocks of proteins. When your body digests protein, it uses those amino acids to manufacture the 50,000 different proteins it needs. It will convert protein into neurotransmitters and chromosomes, hormones and enzymes, antibodies and muscles, hair and nails.

Your body's proteins are made from combinations of just 22 different amino acids. Eight of these are considered essential nutrients for humans and can only be obtained from food. The others can usually be synthesized from the eight and are called 'non-essential', but they are equally vital to life. Because of the importance of amino acids to all the cells in your body, your brain can be at a disadvantage. If your amino acid levels are low, then a competition takes place. Brain cells compete with body cells, which have an advantage because they can take up essential amino acids more easily from your bloodstream. Neurotransmitters are synthesized within your neurons, so their production depends on which amino acids actually get into your brain.

In a study funded by Durham Local Education Authority, the Dyslexia Research Trust, Oxford University and the Dyspraxia Foundation, 120 underachieving children are to be given supplements of refined fish oil, evening primrose and vitamin E. The supplement, called Eye Q, contains high levels of unsaturated omega-3 fatty acids that the brain needs for proper myelination. Disorders of fatty acid metabolism may be a factor in pre-disposing a child to dyslexia, dyspraxia and ADHD.

Another British study has found that one in four schoolgirls studied are damaging their IQs by dieting and depriving themselves of iron.[97] 'We were surprised that a very small drop in iron levels caused a fall in IQ,' explained Dr Michael Nelson, study author and senior lecturer in nutrition at King's College, London. 'We conclude that poor iron status is common among British adolescent girls and diet and iron status play an important role in determining IQ, independent of factors such as menstrual status or social class. By supplementing their diets with extra iron, it is quite probable that cognitive function would improve.'

The researchers surveyed 595 girls, aged 11 to 18, attending three comprehensive schools in North London, making up a cross-section of racial groups. The girls provided blood samples that were assessed for haemoglobin and packed cell volume. The investigators found that there was a highly significant difference in IQ between iron-deficient anaemic girls (with the lowest levels of iron in their blood), iron-deficient and iron-replete girls. Although the study only examined adolescent girls, 'there is also some evidence that people over 65 suffer from lack of iron and cognitive function but this is also linked to deficiencies of folic acid, zinc and vitamin B12'.

Skipping breakfast leads to deterioration in academic performance. In a process known as metabolic starvation, focused attention, recall and coping with complex mental tasks becomes increasingly more difficult. Many UK schools organize breakfast clubs for all children. Cocoa, milk, cereal and toast are low-cost, high-return investments for the schools. Children behave better and learn better. Some research found that those who had eaten a bowl of cereal on the morning of an exam appeared to perform better than children who had eaten no, or an inappropriate, breakfast.

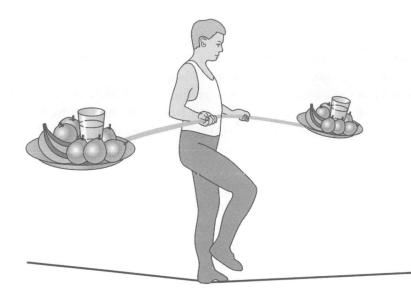

8.1 Children's lifestyles, exercise and diet play their part in shaping the brain they inherit as adults. One in five adults in the UK are obese. Balance is important in all things: physical and intellectual challenge, nutrition, hydration, sleep and fun.

Research at Northumbria University suggested that supplements of ginseng and ginkgo biloba helped improve performance at memory tasks.[98] However, research published in July 2001 by the same university in north-east England showed that chewing gum in exams helped improve performance. When control groups with chewing gum were tested against those without, there was a slight lift in performance. Control groups with no gum but who were asked to simulate chewing for the period of the exam also showed a slight lift in performance. The speculation in this case is that the movement of the jaw contributes to improved oxygen circulation in the head and release of saliva, associated with a state of being relaxed!

Work done on memory and diet by Swansea University found increased errors in memorizing word lists among those skipping breakfast.[99] There were improvements after breakfast and improvements were also connected to the basic rest activity cycle (BRAC). Dr Green at Unilever found that weight loss diets produced impaired functions of memory but the coincident preoccupation with food avoidance was a contributory factor. Babies' brains are permanently impaired by malnutrition during sensitive periods.

Obesity is a growing problem in the West. New evidence suggests that it takes 10 minutes before the brain realizes that the body has taken in enough food. A study carried out at the University of Florida found that the delay in eating and realizing that you are full can lead some people to have an extra portion of pie without realizing they have actually had more than enough.[100] The time the brain takes to respond to glucose ingestion is longer in the obese people than that in normal lean people. The findings are helping to improve the diagnosis and treatment of obesity and other eating disorders.

Brain activity was studied in 18 participants. These people fasted for 12 hours and then underwent continuous brain scanning for 48 minutes. Using fMRI (functional magnetic resonance imaging – a technique for imaging brain activity using magnets), the researchers were able to record the brain's activity in response to internal and external stimuli such as eating and drinking. Ten minutes after the scanning began, participants were given a water solution containing dextrose, a type of sugar. The researchers detected two peaks in brain response after the water solution was taken. The first occurred about 90 seconds afterwards and was, the scientists said, related to swallowing and other aspects of the eating process. The second, more important and sustained peak, began about 10 minutes after the ingestion and was the brain's signal that it was physically full.

The peak lasted about two minutes and corresponded directly with an increase in sugar and insulin levels in the blood. The scientists also identified that the brain changes occurred in the hypothalamus, a portion of the brain responsible for regulating body temperature and metabolism. Yijun Liu, Assistant Professor at the University of Florida's Department of Psychiatry, said the findings may help to develop new drugs to treat obesity and obesity-related diabetes and pointed out which areas of the brain were involved.

‘ The hypothalamus has been known for many years as being related to the regulation of eating. But this is the first study in humans able to directly demonstrate that it undergoes dynamic and physiological changes as a result. ’

It reinforces your mother's advice, which she got from her mother, not to 'bolt' your food. Eating more slowly may provide more time for the feeling of fullness to occur, especially in the obese, whose fullness signals are slower and weaker. One in five adults in the UK is deemed to be obese.

The water solution

If you visit www.urbanlegends.com, one of the myths you will find there is that you must drink at least 2.5 litres of water daily – with an ordinary standard being one millilitre for every calorie of food. The site goes on to explain that this information can be traced to a 1945 edict from the US Academy of Sciences on recommended daily allowances. The last sentence says that most of the water is 'contained in prepared foods'. This last sentence has somehow got lost. Yet many UK schools are restoring water fountains to classrooms and to corridors and many report positive gains as a result of doing so.

At the time of writing, in many, perhaps most, UK primary schools the only source of readily accessible water for children is located in the toilets. Many schools report that allowing children to bring in sports bottles that can then be filled during the day has contributed to improvements in learning performance. While this should not necessarily be taken at face value, it is worth exploring further.

Where do I begin? According to a leaflet given to me on a transatlantic crossing I need 1.5 litres for an 11-hour flight. According to the popular press I need 2 litres a day. According to my mother it is 4 litres and according to The British Dietetic Association currently it is six to eight cups or glasses of water, tea, coffee, juice, or sugar-free drinks per day. David Oliviera of the Department of Renal Medicine at St George's Hospital in London is of the view that

> The minimum volume of urine required by the kidneys to excrete waste products of metabolism is about half a litre per day. Since we lose another half litre via sweat,

breathing and faeces, the net intake required to maintain water balance is about one litre a day under normal conditions. Drinking more than this simply results in more dilute urine – the same absolute amount of toxins will still be excreted.[10]

So if you want your learners to have dilute urine, pile on the water! Dehydration, combined with irregular intake of fluids, combined with fuelling with high concentrate sugar drinks often laced with additives and preservatives may prove a deadly cocktail for the young learners in a classroom. Here are the benefits identified by the international bottled water organization of appropriate intake of fresh water:

- The brain is 75 per cent water so that even moderate dehydration can cause headaches and dizziness.
- Water is required for expiration.
- Regulates body temperature.
- Carries nutrients and oxygen to all cells in the body.
- Blood is 92 per cent water.
- Moistens oxygen for breathing.
- Protects and cushions vital organs.
- Helps to convert food into energy.
- Helps body absorb nutrients.
- Removes waste.
- Bones are 22 per cent water.
- Muscles are 75 per cent water.
- Cushions joints.

Some have argued that the effect of being allowed to drink water as and when it is needed might in itself be a positive thing. Perhaps having a physical reprieve from focused attention in classroom learning in order to visit the water fountain may also be a good thing. Simply having water present may also have a therapeutic value. It does seem that the presence of individual sports-type bottles with fresh water individualizes water intake choice for classroom learners. This self-regulation may be at the heart of the successes schools report. The practical experience of many UK schools sits alongside recent research that suggests drinking it in the right circumstances is very important.

Experimental psychologist Dr Peter Rogers and his colleagues from the University of Bristol carried out tests on 60 volunteers.[102] The volunteers were asked to rate how thirsty they felt. Their reactions were then tested by getting them to press a button in response to prompts on a computer screen. The volunteers either drank nothing before the test or had a cupful (330 millilitres) of tap water, chilled to 10°C. People who were thirsty at the beginning of the test and took a drink performed 10 per cent better than those who drank nothing. But the performance of those who were not thirsty to start with dropped by 15 per cent after a drink.

Dr Rogers believes that drinking too much water might affect the ability to drive or perform intellectually demanding tasks. He thinks that the temperature of the drinks might explain part of the effect. The body has to divert physiological resources to deal with the local cooling effect in the gut and this may be responsible for the effect on performance. The team served the water moderately cold and speculated that perhaps colder, or hot ones would have a greater detrimental impact, and body temperature water the least.

Sleep, learning and the brain

Is there a correlation with academic performance and sleep patterns? According to Dr Larry Cahill of the University of California at Irvine 'learning which is accompanied by some emotional arousal and directed attention, followed by REM sleep is the best form of learning'.[103] So, does sleep improve memory? Can the right sort of sleep pattern make you a better learner? Should I give you time to sleep on it before you answer these questions? The scientific community seems split on the value of findings of research into sleep, learning and memory.[104]

When we sleep, the production of norepinephrine and serotonin is switched off. During the day these chemicals play a part in regulating our logical and consequential thinking, reminding us of time, duration and location. When we are asleep anything goes. Judgement of time and location is distorted. Logic disappears and we drift through 90 to 100 minute cycles of rapid eye movement or REM sleep. REM sleep is a phase characterized by very quick flickering of the eyes and higher levels of brain activity. Typically REM sleep occurs four times throughout the night and is interspersed with non-REM or NREM sleep.

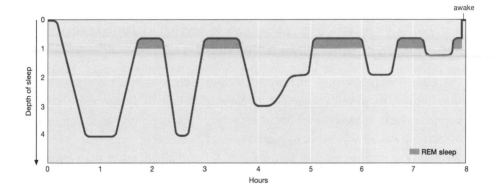

8.2 The stages of rapid eye movement or REM sleep. We spend 20 to 30 per cent of each night in REM sleep, dreaming an average of two hours a night. Within 30 to 45 minutes of falling asleep a deep phase occurs. Then a shallower phase of REM sleep occurs. Towards the end of the night the REM phases become more frequent with periods of deep sleep shorter in duration.

Pierre Maquet of the University of Liège in Belgium suggests that the most likely hypothesis we have is one of consolidation.[105] 'The memory probably isn't actually formed in REM sleep. It's already there, but it seems that the memory is consolidated during REM sleep. Before it's fragile; after, it's more robust.' His team found that brain activity during REM sleep was similar to that recorded by PET scans during a simple keyboarding task completed while awake earlier that day.

Professor Horne at the Sleep Research Laboratory, Loughborough University, looked at sleep deprivation and found impairment of activity within the pre-frontal cortex and reduction in logical thought, impaired choice of words, and reduction in behavioural flexibility, 'All the functions of our body have circadian rhythms [a 24-hour cycle]:'[106]

According to Daniel Kripke, Professor of Psychiatry, UC San Diego, many teenagers, particularly boys in late adolescence, suffer from what is known as sleep delay syndrome.[107] It can begin in puberty and worsens in the late teens. The sleepy phase of the body clock shifts around so that such teenagers cannot get to sleep, cannot get up, are tired all day (especially in the afternoons) and the earlier that school, college or work begins the less sleep they have. What can get truncated is the REM phase of the sleep cycle. Cut across it and what we are left with is a teenager who may be moody, irascible and slightly ill-tempered. Some 2.5 per cent of boys in their late teens in the USA are said to be suffering from this condition!

Professor Robert Stickgold at Harvard Medical School conducted research into procedural memory involving a physical activity.[108] Performance on computer tasks improved after about an hour of practice and then began to plateau. It was only after six or more hours of subsequent sleep that there were marked improvements in performance. But not all phases of sleep have the same value to memory and to learning. To find out exactly what was going on participants were observed in a sleep laboratory. It was discovered that consolidation was optimized when two types of sleep – REM and slow-wave – occurred during the course of the night. Professor Stickgold concludes that a good sleep is important after intensive studying or training because it is during extended deep sleep with oscillations between REM and slow-wave in roughly 90-minute cycles that consolidation of procedural memory occurs.

Others go further in their claims for the significance of findings about brain activity during sleep. Professor Jan Born of Lubeck University, Germany says that, 'certain structures in the brain are active during learning and it shows that during sleep there is a kind of reactivation of these structures. It's beyond doubt that sleep helps to consolidate memories.'[109] He does, however, add a cautionary note, 'the question remains what causes these effects, what mechanisms are responsible? I don't think we are any nearer an answer.' His own work points to slow-wave sleep as essential for learning, with REM sleep having an 'additive effect'. During sleep we alternate between slow-wave and REM. Slow-wave is essential before and after learning new skills and REM consolidates memories of what has been learned.

Anyone who has had a baby knows that sleep deprivation is the oldest and cheapest form of torture. Missing out on sleep too often is dangerous. Not only does this lead to impairment and death of hippocampal cells, but also to injury and death from the accidents caused by sleepy drivers and machine operators each year. Researchers at Harvard Medical School found that cheating on sleep for only a few nights increased brain levels of cortisol. Inadequate sleep also deprived the brain of the time it needs to re-establish its energy. In one survey it was suggested that about two-thirds of the population fail to get enough sleep. With very young children lack of sufficient uninterrupted sleep causes behaviour problems. A study of 500 children under five years of age found that those who slept less than 10 hours a day, including naps, were 25 per cent more likely to misbehave. They would throw temper tantrums, act aggressively to others, be more vocal in their attention seeking and more demanding of adult attention. Children who slept 12 or more hours a day were much less likely to behave in this way.[110]

Kripke has done work on perceived morning sleepiness on at least four mornings per week among 13 year olds and found it varies by country.[111]

Country	%
Norway	45
Finland	40
USA	38
Scotland	35
England	22

All animals operate on rhythms of biological regulation. Humans have highs and lows for different types of physiological and intellectual function and we have 'downtime' through sleep. There is no simple reason for sleep to be necessary. It does not rest the brain, in fact, some parts of the brain are more active in sleep than when we are awake. Circadian rhythms apply to many of our bodily functions. A circadian rhythm is basically a 24 hour cycle. We have three versions of a period gene and they recur throughout the body. Our body clocks are inaccurate – they tend to get later – and can be influenced by things like artificial light. Older people all have different sleep patterns to teenagers and those in their early twenties. The presence of neurotransmitters and brain receptors varies by time of day. It is true to say that some of us are early birds and some are night owls!

Natural births peak at around 5.00am in the morning. There are two peaks for induced labour: one hour before midday and one hour after. The death rate from natural causes is known to be highest at 4.00am. There is so much coming and going in that narrow one-hour window in the early hours of the morning. There are bodily changes too: more cortisol in our bodies at the beginning and at the end of sleep, more growth hormone early in the sleep period. My suggestion would be – give yourself a good lie-in!

Movement, play and learning

How important is play to your child or to the children you teach in your school? British anthropologists Iona and Peter Opie spent years observing children's play. They thought that play, perhaps more than any other aspect of a child's life, was where children learned from their peers. They observed that 'if the present day child was wafted back to any previous century, he would probably find himself at home with the games being played than with any other social custom'.[112] This was written in Britain in 1969. Have things changed?

Perhaps some of the games children play in the playgrounds and the streets of the twenty-first century differ from those of their parents and grandparents, but many games will, nevertheless, retain echoes of things past. The purpose of play is, I believe, consistent and it may well go beyond the transmission of rules and learning of social interactions. When young children are absorbed in play, it becomes more important to them at that time than any other aspect of their lives. I remember my mother's vain attempts to call me in from the field in the midst of some nail-biting finale to a soccer match. As well as being fun, play can be dangerous. Some 80 per cent of deaths among young fur seals occur when playing pups do not recognize the advance of a predator. It can also be exhilarating, energy consuming and is an integral part of being human. Young children use as much as 15 per cent of their total available energy in play. This figure represents a very high commitment to a primate in its developing stage. What is the purpose? A compelling case is made by behavioural scientists that not only does play improve the physique of the youngster in preparation for the rigours of an adult life and help with practising the skills related to hunting, social groupings and mating, but it also gives them bigger, and thus better, brains.

Research published in 2001 suggested that in primates, the amount the brain grows between birth and maturity reflects the amount of play in which each species engages.[113] Earlier studies also suggested a link between general playfulness and brain size. Evolutionary scientist Robert Barton believes it has to do with preparation for learning and probably, 'with the importance of environmental input to the neo-cortex and to the cerebellum during development.'[114] The process of synaptogenesis involves the overproduction of connections between neurons in sensitive periods of a primate's development. In other words your brain produces more connections than it needs but only for a short window of time. During this window the extent to which connections are laid down depends on the duration and level of stimulation the brain receives. Animals, young humans specifically, can sculpt the overall circuitry of the brain through play. They lay down the neural pathways needed later in life. Neuroscientist Dr Steven Siviy studied how play affected the chemicals in the brain and in particular proteins associated with the stimulation and growth of nerve cells. He found that play activated lots of different areas of the brain and could play a part not only in learning but in creativity.[115]

Young children who are imaginative in their make-believe play are better able to cope with stress later in life, according to another contemporary US-based research project.[116] Creative five and six year olds often end up better problem solvers by the time they are nine and ten. 'Good early play skills predicted the ability to be creative and generate alternative solutions to everyday problems,' said researcher Sandra W. Russ, Professor and Chair of the Psychology Department at Case Western Reserve University.

The children in the study were given three types of creativity tests: Affect in Fantasy Task, an Alternate Uses Test, and a Story Telling Measure. In the first test the children were asked to make up a play using two puppets and three blocks. The Alternate Uses Test measured divergent thinking – thinking that explores various solutions to a problem. In the Story Telling Measure, the children were asked to make up a story to go along with a picture book for younger children.

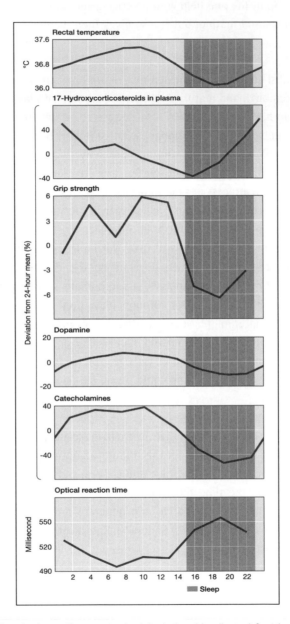

8.3 Circadian rhythms affect many physiological and intellectual functions. Seen here are body temperature and grip strength changes, optical reaction times and alterations in the chemicals cortisol, dopamine and catecholamine. Notice how in there is a flat period followed by a rise towards the end of the sleep phase.

It was discovered that the processes learned in pretend play are important because they relate to adaptive functioning in children – creativity abilities, coping abilities. To foster creativity in children, the researchers suggest:

- ▶ allowing time to indulge in play.

- ▶ participating with children as they play.

- ▶ praising and rewarding children for their creativity and imagination.

- ▶ helping children if they need suggestions for creative play.

Play excites different parts of the brain. Children's play can simultaneously excite auditory, visual, motor and spatial functions. When young children are encouraged in learning to explore through their senses, separate areas of the motor cortex and sensory motor cortex are activated. The motor and sensory motor strip runs across the top of the brain left and right like an Alice band. In the human brain larger areas of the cortex are devoted to movements such as thumb and forefinger and the muscles around the mouth and the manipulation of the tongue.

Research with adults has shown that exercises using delicate finger movements will, within days, be rewarded with more sensory real estate being devoted to those functions.[117] Rats have large areas of the sensory strip devoted to the manipulation of the whiskers. The rats use their whiskers to explore and find out about their world. Children explore and find out about their world through play. Through sensory interaction the structure of the motor and sensory motor strip changes. The best learning is like play.

Play involves lots of rehearsal and repetition. Children do things again and again. It can, and most often does, involve stepped levels of challenge and of risk. There is an engagement at an emotional level and later at different social levels. Play is not something the contemporary Western child is given opportunity for or learns as of right. With more and more children driven to and picked up from neighbourhood schools, sat in front of televisions or computer games and losing the skills of co-operative play learned by their grandparents, maybe it is time to start teaching children how to play?

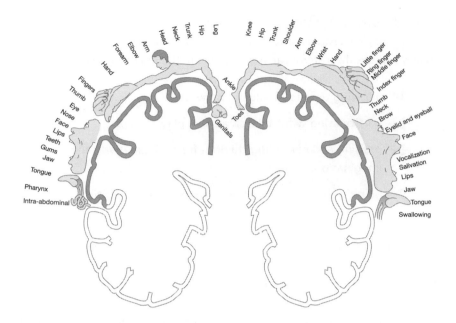

8.4 The homunculus or 'little man' is a graphical illustration of the sensitivity and function of the motor and sensory areas of the cerebral cortex. The motor cortex is located like an Alice band across the top of the head between the ears. The diagram represents the region of the body that moves following stimulus of that part of the cortex. Notice how very sensitive areas like the hands, mouth and lips have more cortical space devoted to them.

In the UK, schoolchildren currently sit an average of 75 external tests designed to assess academic aptitude. There is increasing pressure to get more and more 'academic' content knowledge into smaller and smaller periods of time. One of the experiences getting squeezed is that of structured physical exercise. Yet, much research of worth points to the benefits for academic performance that regular physical exercise gives. Angela Balding of Exeter University looked at the activity levels of secondary age pupils in the UK and found that regular exercise could be correlated to improvements in academic performance.[118] More than 1,400 children took part in the research. 'We found a definite link between those youngsters who exercise at least three or four times a week and those who did better in the classroom,' said Balding. She then suggested a possibility that 'the kids who are active get more oxygen to their brains more often. As a result their brains could be more receptive to learning new information and retaining it.'

The early indications of a three-year research project begun in April 1999 by the UK Qualifications and Curriculum Authority with 30 schools found that those with a high participation in sports tend to have lower truancy rates and less bad behaviour. Coincidental research by Sport England in 1999 showed that the amount of sport played in primary schools has been reduced by a third in the period 1994 to 1999.

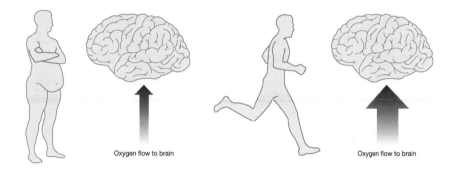

Oxygen flow to brain   Oxygen flow to brain

8.5   The more efficient the system, the more agile it becomes. Oxygen uptake to the brain is improved by structured physical activity.

The adult brain, although only about 2 per cent of body weight, receives 16 per cent of the blood supply and per unit mass brain tissue receives ten times as much blood as muscle tissue. By the age of three the brain is 80 per cent of adult size and by the age of five the brain is 90 per cent of adult size. In adults about 25 per cent of the oxygen in the system is used by the brain and in young children it is nearer 50 per cent. Professor Susan Greenfield of Oxford University, one of the world's leading authorities on the brain, says that 'the brain is very sensitive to what is happening to the body and the more you are interacting and stimulating the circuits of the brain, the more agile are your brain cells'. In the Exeter Fit to Succeed Project more than 60 per cent of 11-year-old boys who achieved level five – above average for the age group – in their maths had taken part in hard physical exercise on at least three occasions in the previous week. Case proven.

You've got to laugh about it

In 1982 I was working as a museum guide in the Lake District in the UK. My job involved telling groups of tourists about the literary associations of the area. I worked within a museum and would take as many as 12 tours a day each lasting 40 minutes. I had been a student, I was not well off and so I worked long hours seven days a week. One morning, midway through a sentence about Wordsworth's poetic method, I got a fit of the giggles. Nothing too extraordinary had happened. I had noticed the gardener, who doubled as the chief museum guide, wander by the window. As he did so he looked in and pulled a face. I fell about laughing and could not stop. As 14 bemused Japanese tourists looked on, I laughed and laughed. Eventually I had to give up the tour and go home for the day. My involuntary and uncontrollable laughing 'fit' had been my mechanism for relieving the physical stress of work.

In 1962 in Tanzania, a girls' school closed after an outbreak of laughter. The outbreak spread beyond the school's gates and within weeks had appeared in the villages where the girls lived. Approximately 10,000 people were affected. Laughter can be hysterical!

There is a lot of research into laughter. In December 2001 the world's funniest joke was named. In research devised in collaboration with the British Association for the Advancement of Science, the University of Hertfordshire, UK, created a website for visitors to submit and rate jokes called the 'Laughlab'.[119] With over 10,000 jokes submitted from over 70 countries, the 'Laughlab' is described as the world's most extensive psychology experiment ever. Over 100,000 people rated the jokes and, in doing so, told the researchers a lot about differences between male and female humour and about national differences. The interim findings showed that males favour more aggressive jokes, jokes with sexual innuendo and jokes at the expense of women. Women prefer jokes with word play. The top joke of all was this one: The famous detective Sherlock Holmes and his partner Dr Watson go camping, and pitch their tent under the stars. During the night Holmes wakes his companion and says: 'Watson, look up at the stars and tell me what you deduce.' Watson says, 'I see millions of stars and, even if only a few of those have planets, it's quite likely that there are some planets like Earth and, if there are a few planets like Earth out there, there might also be life.' Holmes replies: 'Watson you idiot. Somebody stole our tent.'

There is also research into laughter and learning. Laughter in a classroom can be a very positive way to reduce stress and aid learning. Laughter, when it precedes certain types of problem solving, improves our general performance. We become more able to deal with cognitive challenge when we approach the challenge having shared laughter with others. Laughter also changes our physical state. It contributes to enhancing the immune system, increasing natural disease fighting cells. It lowers levels of immunosuppressive hormones while, at the same time, boosting white blood cells. It lowers blood pressure and has a beneficial effect on conditions such as cancer and rheumatoid arthritis. It can reduce the symptoms of depression. Laughter is known to relieve stress, improve sleep and produce a general sense of well-being.

In the USA, the American Association for Therapeutic Humor – where the therapy is known as 'hee hee healing' – has commissioned over 100 studies of the beneficial effects of humour. In one study by Dr Jason Goodson of Utah University, patients were given therapeutic tapes of comedians to listen to for 30 minutes a day for four weeks.[120] Using a scoring system, the patients had an average depression score of 19. Anything above 13 is considered mild to moderate depression. After listening to the tapes, the group as a whole dropped to 11. The 42 per cent reduction in symptoms was considered significant. At Christmas 2001 the UK retailer Asda, owned by Wal-Mart, replaced piped music in its shops with jokes in an attempt to relieve customer stress and keep them in the shops longer. With 11 million visitors to UK stores in the week before Christmas, Asda were playing for big stakes. This is one of the jokes the customers heard: 'Who is never hungry at Christmas?' Answer: 'The turkey – he's always stuffed!'

Roll on Easter!

Researchers struggle to explain what is happening in the brain when we laugh. It is understood to be an instinctive response programmed by our genes. Identical twins reared apart for 40 years had identical laughs. Individuals who are autistic have great difficulty in understanding humour. They experience things literally. Laughter has a social function. Laughter provokes more laughter: you laugh with others and so it is good for relationships. If you tickle yourself, you do not laugh – why? It has a social dimension – studies have shown that people are 30 times more likely to laugh in social settings than when alone. Even nitrous oxide loses much of its potency when taken in solitude. Extroverts (people who are outgoing) prefer sexual and simple jokes, while introverts (people who are shy) prefer non-sexual and more complicated jokes. *You Laugh, You Lose!* was the name of an American TV show where contestants had to avoid laughing or smiling for one full minute to win $200. The show was abandoned because the audience laughed a lot but the contestants did not.

You laugh in preferred ways – just like you learn: some people find visual jokes funny, others find auditory jokes funny and others like physical (or kinesthetic) jokes. People laugh in similar but not identical fashion, often in variations of five notes. You often get:

Ha ha ha ha ha
Ho ho ho ho ho
He he he he he

You never get:

Ha ho ha ho ha
He ho he ho he

Research shows that males are better at getting laughs but females are better at laughing. It also suggests that people who giggle a lot are less likely to get jobs. Young children laugh on average up to 300 times daily, adults 25 to 30 times.

Sing when you are winning

At soccer matches in the UK it is common to hear fans sing in support of their team. This is assumed by social commentators to be a form of tribalism which helps the sporting performance of the players on the field. Examples of popular favourites include 'You'll Never Walk Alone', 'There's Only One Man

United' and 'Who is the Authority Figure of Questionable Parentage Wearing a Black Outfit running around in the Centre?' Another all-time terracing hit – 'Sing When You Are Winning, You Only Sing When You Are Winning ...' – is now known to have literal as well as metaphorical truth. Singing raises the level of antibodies produced by the body.

Research by the University of California at Irvine showed how singing can produce physical and emotional benefits.[121] Using cotton swabs to collect saliva from the mouths of 32 choristers who had just sung a Beethoven piece, the team showed that immunoglobulin A levels had gone up dramatically. Immunoglobulin A (IgA) is used by the body's immune system to fight off disease. During rehearsals levels of IgA increased by 150 per cent and in performance by 240 per cent. In the study, the authors – Professor Robert Beck and Dr Tom Cesario – point out that 'secretory immunoglobulin protein is associated with emotional arousal and mood, relaxation and sense of humour. If singing leads to higher levels of IgA, then it is beneficial to your health as we know that heightened levels of this protein are effective in the immune system.' Singing releases endorphins, it alters your breathing, it stimulates the nerves behind the stomach. Singing together is a good form of team building. Earlier we showed how learning through music helps children remember related content. So, the class that sings together, wins together!

Chapter 9

Engagement:

how do we arouse and direct the brain?

This chapter contains the following sections:

⚖ **Stress, learning and the brain**
A definition of stress. The physical changes that come about as a result of stress.

⚖ **Dangerous dimensions of stress**
Glucocorticoids. Good and bad ways to prepare for exams. How stress makes it difficult to create new memories.

⚖ **Dealing with stressors**
What to do to deal with stress. How rats and humans share stress responses. Classroom tools for dealing with learner stress.

⚖ **The four 'F's of classroom survival**
Challenge and stress: a vital difference to a learner. What happens to a classroom learner under stress? A summary of likely behavioural responses and what to do about each.

⚖ **Get yourself engaged**
Emotions and their origin. How we all have different emotional palettes. Emotional adaptability and susceptibility.

⚖ **A motivational model**
A little more about motivation followed by a seven-stage motivational model.

... and will answer the following questions:

- In what ways might stress get in the way of learning? How does challenge differ from stress?

- If I get stressed, what happens to my body?

- How do we know so much about stress?

- How can I recognize a learner under stress? What can I do once I recognize the stress responses?

- What is the difference between engaged and disengaged emotions?

- I feel apathetic. Have you got something that will help me think my way out of a rut?

Introduction

In the last year, have you ever been stressed? Did your stress extend beyond the immediate moment? Did you feel out of control and unable to do anything about it? Did it affect your relationships? Appetite? General health? Energy levels? Enthusiasm for work?

If you answered yes to any or all of these, welcome to what being an adult in the West in the twenty-first century has become about. Adults in the West in our time no longer die in great numbers of malaria, liver fluke, dysentery, leprosy or tuberculosis. They do, however, die of stress-related illnesses such as diabetes, cancer, strokes and ulcers. We have become accomplished at turning on the stress response. We are not so gifted at turning it off.

Professor Robert Sapolsky is a primatologist who specializes in glucocorticoids (a class of steroid hormones secreted from the adrenal glands – and more commonly known as cortisol). He has spent years in the company of baboons. He gives wonderfully illustrated talks on stress in large primates. He compares the physical changes evidenced by stress in baboons with those evidenced in humans. He starts his talks by pointing out how, in the West, we have slowly accumulated dysfunction over time including the luxury of dying from stress-related illness.[122]

Stress, learning and the brain

A stressor is defined as anything from the outside world that puts us out of homeostatic balance. We can do this through thought and if we do it chronically, we will get sick. The stress response is anything we do to restore the homeostatic balance. We can do this through thought and if we do it well enough, we will recover. Professor Sapolsky affirms that we can turn on the stress response simply by thought but asks, 'Are we smart enough to turn it off?'

Your sympathetic nervous system mobilizes you to deal with threat, real or imagined. Your adrenal glands release adrenaline (also known as epinephrine) and other hormones that increase breathing, heart rate and blood pressure.

This moves more oxygen-rich blood faster to the brain and to the muscles needed for fighting or fleeing. Adrenaline causes a rapid release of glucose and fatty acids into your bloodstream to give you energy. Your senses become keener, your memory sharper, and you are less sensitive to pain.

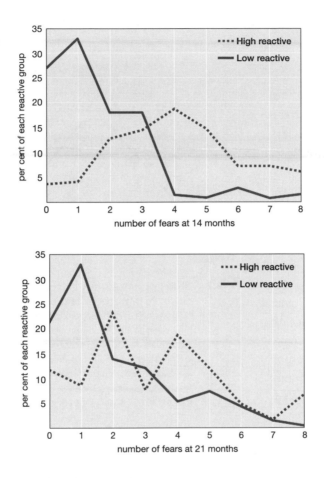

9.1 The charts show how young children cope differently to stress based on temperament and life experience. In each age range a set of physiological responses to an event that could be construed as 'fearful' was measured. Some children showed little or no reaction. Others were more disposed to demonstrate a stress response. Children who were deemed 'high reactives' at 14 months were also found to be more susceptible to 'fearful' events at 21 months and at 48 months.

Other functions shut down while all this is going on. While struggling for survival you do not want to grow, have sex or eat and blood flow to the skin is reduced. That is why chronic stress leads to sexual dysfunction, increases your chance of getting sick and gives you a rash or spots. Your body is now in a temporary state of metabolic overdrive and you are prepared to respond to a life-threatening situation. After you have done so and the danger has passed, your body tries to return to normal. It is incredibly easy to turn on the stress response but it is also incredibly difficult to turn it off. Scientists agree that the stress response is predetermined by genes and by childhood experience. It is only voluntary to a limited extent and there is a sub-set of people who, for some unexplained reason, are better than the rest of us at coping with it.

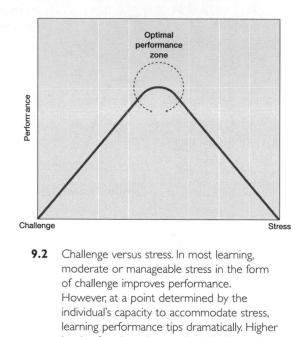

9.2 Challenge versus stress. In most learning, moderate or manageable stress in the form of challenge improves performance. However, at a point determined by the individual's capacity to accommodate stress, learning performance tips dramatically. Higher levels of anxiety characterize this phase. For teachers, balancing challenge with anxiety-related stress is part of their professional skill.

In response to stress the body has any combination of 11 different chemicals to release. It will begin to do so in less than a second of a stressor being identified. What happens is that the excitatory sympathetic nervous system jumps into action immediately, but it is very slow to turn off and allow the inhibitory parasympathetic nervous system to take over and calm you down. Once the stress response has been activated, the system wisely keeps you in a state of readiness: the predator might come back. Keeping it on carries consequences for your health.

Adaptive stress response	Stress-related disorder
Mobilize energy	Fatigue, diabetes
Blood pressure up	Hypertension
Stop eating	Ulceration, colitis
Stop growing	Dwarfism
Stop having sex	Impotency, reduced libido
Suppression of immune system	Increased disease risk
Think faster	Eventual neural degeneration
Sharpening of sensory systems	Death of neurons related to learning and memory

Some stress in learning is good. Maze performance in rats goes up in the short term when they are injected with a stress hormone. It is at the point when a feeling of loss of control and helplessness kicks in that problems arise. This is all too prevalent in everyday life in the West.

For the first hour or so stress helps some types of learning. It helps produce more oxygen to the brain in the short term. Neurons have more energy resource at their disposal. In this stage of engagement we learn better. Sadly, it does not last. After about six hours of this unrelieved stress, short-term memory begins to go.

After about a week, we see the beginnings of atrophy of neural networks. The hippocampus is weakened and begins to show signs of ageing faster. According to Professor Sapolsky, energy is diverted away from the hippocampus and cortex towards the cerebellum. Explicit memory is adversely affected and implicit memory is favoured.

Dangerous dimensions of stress

Your lifestyle will also be affected by stress. The most dangerous set of personality traits to hold onto are those of the type 'A' personality – particularly in men. If you know someone who, habitually, has a negative fixation on life, who exhibits impatience and joylessness, have a word. Remaining so will affect their diet, their immune system, their growth, their sleep and their ability to have children. The worst trait is the combination of hostility with impatience.

The bacteria contributing to stomach ulcers multiply faster in stress. Your immune system is less effective so you are more susceptible to disease. Testosterone levels in males go down as does their capacity to reproduce. According to Sapolsky, choir boys in the Vatican have higher levels of testosterone than young American marines going through boot camp. With excess of exercise and the subsequent stress, athletes stop ovulating. You do not eat, nor do you grow. Stress-related dwarfism, although extremely rare, does occur. Get a child out of stress and he starts to grow again.

To understand how stress impacts on learning and how some children fall victim to the stress response that will limit their learning before they ever get to a classroom, you must know about cortisol.

Sustained stress can damage the hippocampus, the part of our limbic system central to learning, spatial recall and memory. The presence of 'glucocorticoids' during stress for longer than they remain useful is the problem. During a perceived threat, your adrenal glands immediately release adrenaline. After a couple of minutes, if the threat is severe or still persists, the adrenals then release cortisol.

Once in the brain, cortisol remains much longer than adrenaline and continues to affect brain cells. Too much adversely affects brain function, especially memory. Human studies show a correlation between high cortisol levels and decreased memory and cognitive functions like concentration and creativity. Learning and memory is all about long-term potentiation (LTP) in the hippocampus. LTP means neurons being better able to communicate with each other. Hippocampal neurons are vulnerable. They get older faster. Months of stress will kill off hippocampal neurons outright. Post Traumatic Stress Disorder, sustained depression and extended sexual abuse in childhood can have a similar effect on the hippocampus.

Highly stressed revision such as the cramming favoured by adolescents, particularly boys, contributes to short-term loss of memory. In a controlled experiment, researchers at the Washington University School of Medicine gave high doses of cortisol to a group of volunteers, while another group received a placebo. After four days the group that had taken the high dose of cortisol showed a significantly lower ability to memorize a written passage.[123] The effect is reversible. After a week off cortisol, the volunteers found memory quickly returned to normal.

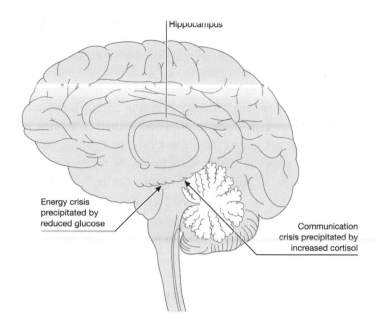

9.3 Stress, cortisol and learning. The hippocampus is increasingly affected by stress chemicals. It becomes less efficient at memory creation. Connections between neurons are also less efficient and long-term potentiation (LTP) becomes more difficult.

The timing of the stressful experience and its severity also correlates to a drop in memory performance. Thirty minutes after rats were stressed by an unanticipated electrical shock, they were unable to remember their way around a maze. When the shock was given two minutes or four hours before going through the maze, the rats had no problem. This time-dependent effect on memory performance correlates with the levels of cortisol circulating in the system, which are highest at 30 minutes. The same thing happened when non-stressed rats were injected with cortisol. When cortisol production was chemically suppressed, there were no stress-induced effects on memory retrieval. The effect only lasts for a couple of hours, so that the impairing effect in this case is a temporary impairment of retrieval. The memory is not lost, it is just inaccessible or less accessible for a period of time.

The presence of excess cortisol affects brain function in two ways. First, because stress hormones divert blood glucose to exercising muscles, the amount of glucose – hence energy – that reaches the hippocampus is diminished. This creates an energy crisis in the hippocampus that makes it unable to create new memories. That is why some people cannot remember a very traumatic event, and why short-term memory is usually the first casualty of age-related memory loss. As we age, it becomes more difficult to turn off the stress response. We take longer to adjust and the sensors in our blood vessels become less efficient at telling us our blood pressure is back to normal. Second, as mentioned earlier, cortisol interferes with the function of neurotransmitters, the chemicals that brain cells use to communicate with each other. This leads to people experiencing difficulty in thinking or accessing long-term memories. It is why they become befuddled and confused in a severe crisis – 'the lines are down' and thus the mind goes blank.

Dealing with stressors

So what can we do to modify stress in ourselves, our children and in our classrooms? First, we need to identify what the causes of stress are, acknowledge that the stress response varies by individual and do what we can to help those individuals manage the stressors in their lives. This is where laboratory research helps. Professor Sapolsky has conducted research with laboratory rats and susceptibility to stress-related disorders such as ulcers.[124] The stressors for rats are like the stressors for humans:

- unpredictability
- sudden surprise
- lack of control over environment
- lack of stimulation in the environment
- no outlet for stress response
- physical inactivity
- no other rats.

When rats are given mild electric shocks on their own with no predictability, their susceptibility to ulcer increases considerably as a result. When shocked in the presence of other rats, they are slightly less susceptible: they can take out their anger on another rat. When, 10 seconds prior to a shock, there is a warning signal there is less stress. Being able to press a lever so that the rat believes it can control or decrease the shock reduces stress. The presence of other rats reduces stress.

The speed with which the rat demonstrates a stress response is also, in part, shaped by the duration of weaning in its immature phase. Rats who were intensely groomed and licked showed more resistance to stressful situations and anxiety as adults. Removing lab rats from their mothers for a few hours a day increased the stress response. It is believed that the stress response is largely set during the period pre-birth to early childhood.

The implications for classroom learning are there for all to see. When we look at the sorts of experiences that cause stress in classroom learning, we find many similarities between Sapolsky's rats and humans. The stressors for learners include:

- unpredictability
- excessive risk
- perceived threat
- lack of feedback
- poor progress measures
- inability to connect to past, present or future needs
- lack of self-belief
- no outlet for stress response
- lack of physical reprieve
- no or little purposeful social interaction.

According to work done by Weiss, Levine and Seligman, the psychological modifiers of the stress response are:[125]

- outlets for frustration
- sense of predictability
- sense of control
- a perception of life improving
- social support.

For a teacher this is a serious message. To overcome stressors build learning challenges onto a familiar framework. Help learners perceive the benefits, know where they are going and how they will get there. Ensure they feel free from intimidation or put-down and are encouraged to negotiate risk. Create a safe haven for managing challenge within your classroom. Create, and celebrate, a sense of collective achievement and every now and again enjoy a laugh together.

The four 'F's of classroom survival

I suggested earlier that all meaningful learning for life involves risk. In circumstances when you 'feel' safe you will be willing to negotiate a higher level of risk. Some of us are risk tolerant and some of us are risk averse with all points between equally represented. If you are in a learning situation and anxiety tips into stress, then what happens next is predictable. There are four categories of survival response available to you. A teacher or anyone who is involved in formally educating others will be familiar with them. They are fight, flight, freeze and flock. You show resistance or fight the source of stress, you flee from it, you freeze in the face of it or you hang out with others like you or flock from it. If you have an accumulation of stressors that leave you feeling out of control, then the four 'F's are what is left for you.

Robert Sapolsky reminds us that the reason a zebra does not get an ulcer is that while it is very good at mobilizing a stress response in the face of threat, it is also very good at turning off the stress response should it survive to be able do so. Humans, particularly adults in the West, are less good at turning off the stress response. The survival options available to a zebra are similar to those available to a child in a classroom: it can flock – hang around with a bunch of other zebras and hope that the hungry lion picks on one of them; it can freeze – merge into the background, stay still, hope the lion goes by; it can flee – get away fast and mobilize all of its running power to outrun the lion; or, last option, it can fight – get power to the big limbs, raise the pain threshold, block out distractions, become intensely focused on beating up that lion.

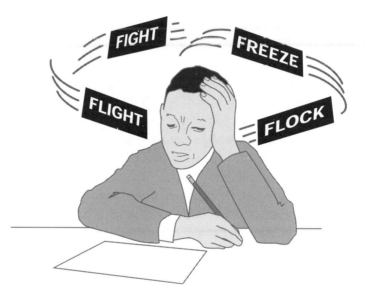

9.4 Learning characterized by high levels of anxiety is one where the four 'F's of survival prevail. Learners who feel intimidated, isolated by a sense of failure, put-down or without control will fight, flight, freeze and flock. They will do so in predictable ways and in combination. They are survival responses.

For a child in a classroom, flocking involves adopting the norms, values and behaviours of the herd – in this case the peer group. The peer group will police and, in some cases, collectively suppress learning performance in a classroom. In these circumstances, the flock or peer group shapes performance and it is difficult to be different. Children will not volunteer ignorance, display enthusiasm or curiosity if they belong to a flock that promotes indifference.

Freezing is the default position when you get stuck or do not know the answer when a question is suddenly thrust at you – it is like temporary paralysis. Teachers who pounce with their questions paralyse performance. Freezing happens when we cannot immediately access a high or low road response. It is like the brain deciding more time is needed for this so let us suspend activity in the interim.

Flight is the use of every avoidance tactic known to schoolchildren the world over, in the hope the teacher engages with someone else. Many children develop skilled classroom avoidance techniques from an early age: they keep their heads down, they do the minimum, they get by. In large classes where the teacher does not know the child, avoidance techniques are more likely to be successful.

Fight is any form of tantrum, rebelliousness, dissent or mock outrage and, in some schools, it is about physical stuff too. When we are in fight mode we resort to deep-seated learned patterns of response. Learned responses come out when we are highly anxious. It is that point when the red mist descends. Overcoming unhelpful learned responses is one of the tools a teacher can bequeath to a child. In the anxiety of an exam I have observed children default to answering English Literature questions on novels they have never read! The learned response was to write – and do as much of it as possible! The default mode in the stress of the exam is get an answer down, get it down quickly and with as much content as possible. As we discussed earlier, learned responses can be altered at a number of levels. Mental rehearsals of positive patterns of behaviour can displace less useful modes.

Get yourself engaged

Novelty engages curiosity. Curiosity engages attention. It is a U-shaped curve. There are only so many times an experience remains new. Novelty, curiosity and attention are all serviced by a range of emotional systems. Separate emotional systems have their own developmental history, their own trigger points for engagement and, within the brain, their own neural assemblies. There is no one centre in the brain that runs all emotional systems. For some emotions, there is a need for them to be present earlier in our development.

It is useful, for survival purposes, to be fearful and this is there early. The startle response is there from the first few days. It is useful for survival purposes to attach oneself to an adult and this is also there early. For other emotions, a more complex developmental history prevails. Anger may emerge from fear and from attachment – maybe – but what survival value does sadness have? Each individual has an emotional palette that is unique to them.

The colours in the emotional palette come about partly as a result of genetic inheritance and partly through our life experiences. The extent to which this palette can be brought successfully to give colour and meaning to everyday experience varies by individual. Some have a range of emotional colours in their palette and the palette ready to hand. Others have few colours in a palette that is awkward to use. Emotional adaptability is a measure of maturity. I will call this an 'engaged emotional response'. It means being able to draw on and manage a range of appropriate emotional responses situation by situation. Emotional susceptibility is a measure of immaturity. I will call this a 'dis-engaged emotional response'. This means as situations change, there are few appropriate emotional responses to draw from. The individual is locked in to patterns from which it is difficult to break free. This may cause further upset, even trauma. This is no judgement on which colours and mix of colours from the emotional palette are best. It is surely healthy to experience fear, sadness, anger, love, joy, loathing, disgust, surprise and guilt. It is not so healthy to be locked in to one of those emotions. When we are in an engaged emotional state, we have colour and shape in our lives. When we are in a disengaged emotional state – in trauma, or depressed or apathetic – we lack colour, shape and, ultimately, choice. In such circumstances, what can be done?

A motivational model

If an individual is clinically depressed, suffering from anxiety attacks, from PTSD (post traumatic stress disorder) or from any condition that is profoundly affecting her ability to make choices in her life, she needs professional help. If an individual needs to feel motivated again, to have a sense of purpose, to connect with a wider range of experiences including emotional experiences, to break free from indifference and feel connected, then learning professionals can help.

Motivation is emotion in motion. Sufficiently motivated, an individual will experience physiological changes. The internal reward system is activated. Different circuitry – the amygdala, the nucleus accumbens, the basal ganglia, the brain stem and the hippocampus – become involved. Research shows that with proper motivation, learning is quicker. More areas of the cortex become involved.

We can link to external reward systems but engaging the internal reward systems is better. How do we do this? By persuading the participant of the benefits. Because we are complex creatures this is not a simple selling job. Some of us are motivated towards success, others away from failure. For some external material or peer reward is best – short term – while for others there is value and pleasure in the experience itself: flow. What follows is a seven-stage motivational model. It is designed to be neutral on which benefits ought to accrue. It can be used individually or with others. Use it if it is useful to you.

Stage one
Conceptualize outcome
What is it you want?

Stage two
Outcome compares favourably when tested against experience
How is what you want better than what you currently have?

Stage three
Outcome capable of mental rehearsal
If you should get what you want, what would it look like? How will you know you have been successful? What will others say to you? How will you feel?

Stage four
Willingness to move to outcome
When will you start to obtain your outcome?

Stage five

Movement secures approval

How will you remind yourself, or let others know, of your outcome?

Stage six

Able to landmark movement to outcome

What will you do first? And then?

Stage seven

Optimism retained throughout process

What will you do to stay positive about your outcome?

To be able and willing to mentally rehearse positive personal outcomes, to conceptualize success – however framed – and to be self-aware throughout is a very useful set of lifelong learning tools to be able to bring to any challenge. To be emotionally resilient enough to accommodate adversity when it does not go right first time is another. You need to be able to complete each stage in turn before graduating to a successor stage. The seven-stage model is one way of helping an individual experience emotional engagement. In the next chapter we look at a different form of brain engagement.

Chapter **10**

Laterality:

how do we develop left and right?

This chapter contains the following sections:

⚏ **Purposeful asymmetry**
The development of left and right difference in the brain.

⚏ **Does the left hand know what the right is doing?**
What makes someone left or right handed. The prevalence of handedness across different cultures.

⚏ **Language and hemisphericity**
How language is generated in the brain. Why some people do not understand jokes. Why others cannot stop telling lies.

⚏ **Stay away from the medicine man**
The emotions and asymmetry. Facts about depression and heart attacks. Classic voodoo death research and why it should be of interest to you.

⚏ **The eyes have it**
How what you believe is not what you see. The cross-lateral design of our optic systems. Japanese reading systems.

⚏ **Listen to me when I'm talking**
Dichotic listening. Does moving the telephone receiver from one ear to another change the way you listen? With which ear do children hear best?

⚏ **So what can we conclude about left and right?**
Challenge and stress: a vital difference to a learner. What happens to a classroom learner under stress. A summary of likely behavioural responses and what to do about each.

✠ **What might this mean for formal learning?**
Too much of the same leads to boredom. Ten suggestions for holistic learning.

... and will answer the following questions:

⇥ How do left/right differences develop in the brain?

⇥ What determines handedness?

⇥ What is so funny about a joke?

⇥ How does a stroke affect the emotions?

⇥ Why does a brain-damaged patient 'see' the world differently?

⇥ Do children have an ear preference?

⇥ What should I know about differences in the left and right sides of my brain?

⇥ How should I organize learning to accommodate hemispheric difference?

Introduction

A man has had a stroke. It has affected the left hemisphere of his brain. This has presented him with some physical problems. Because the adjacent motor control areas in his left hemisphere were damaged, the right side of his body is affected. He has difficulty in smiling. His smile is now lopsided. His speech is slurred and he struggles to move his right hand freely. His wife tells him a joke.

Patient: 'I've just swallowed a pillow.'
Doctor: 'How do you feel?'
Patient: 'A little down in the mouth.'

He hears the joke and laughs. His face lights up, his eyes brighten and both sides of his mouth lift in a natural smile. The implicitly learned, spontaneous laughter response is primed by emotional centres in the brain and not by the motor cortex. Temporarily, the faulty circuitry in the left hemisphere is bypassed.

The difference in function between the left and the right hemispheres has caught popular interest more than any other area of brain research. So much so, that the lines between fallacy, fad and fact are badly blurred. Fuelling this interest has been a strong desire on the part of the self-help movement, and some educators, for a one-line answer. In a well intended desire to seek human integration at all levels, the idea of left and right brain became a working metaphor for educating the whole person. Who can resist

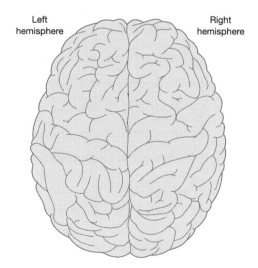

Left hemisphere

Right hemisphere

10.1 The two hemispheres of the human brain are not identical but in all complex tasks both are involved. There are left and right differences in how language is understood and produced and in the computation of spatial relationships. Chemicals to do with emotional arousal and inhibition, selective attention and managing impulsivity differ in their distribution left and right. Male and female brains also differ left and right.

the idea that a re-alignment of education priorities might afford a more 'brain compatible solution' to learning? To this end, a heavy industry of educators emerged who were willing to fulfil the brief of, for example, this UK training programme advertised for teachers in September 2000, 'participants will learn how to teach the right-brained learner.

Meanwhile scientific research, which had long since forgotten to define the brain in such terms and no longer had an explicit focus on hemispheric difference, went on to ask increasingly sophisticated questions to which asymmetry of function remained a fundamental organizing principle. Notions of right and left brain became considerations and not answers. It should be said, there is no gene, no chemical, no neural assembly, no lobe, no region and no hemisphere in the human brain that is singly responsible for any behaviour! Nor is there a chemical or a cell type or a structure that is present in one hemisphere but not in the other. When we understand this we can leave behind forever the fad of the right- or the left-brain learner!

Roger Sperry won the Nobel Prize in Medicine in 1981. Sperry was awarded the prize 'for his discoveries concerning the functional specialization of the cerebral hemispheres'. His work broke new ground in understanding how the human brain is lateralized. In his Nobel acceptance speech in Stockholm, he talked of the significance of some of his work for educators,

> The more we learn, the more we recognize the unique complexity of any one individual intellect, the stronger the conclusion becomes that the individuality inherent in our brain networks makes that of fingerprints or facial features gross and simple by comparison.[126]

He went on to suggest a need for recognizing such individuality, 'The need for educational tests and policy measures to identify, accommodate and serve the differentially specialized forms of individual intellectual potential becomes increasingly evident.' Sperry died in 1984. Work on left and right brain was colonized by the media, by the self-help movement and eventually by some educators and now has a residual metaphoric status. People describe themselves as 'very right brained'. What this now means is creative, slightly disorganized, eccentric and forgivably wacky. No one ever admits to being left brained but, if they did, it would be code for dull, plodding, predictable and ever so slightly and unforgivably anal. I did a quick search on Amazon Books website to find out how many popular science books they sold with the words 'right and left brain' somewhere in the title. Result? Forty-seven. There is obviously enormous interest and some scholarship in this field, so what do we know and what does the current understanding of right and left brain tell us about human learning?

Purposeful asymmetry

There is much virtue in having a body that is symmetrical. If you have a limb torn off by a sabre tooth tiger, then you have another limb that looks and performs much the same to compensate. You can get on with being a hunter-gatherer or do a bit of compensatory foraging instead. Provided you survive the trauma, the loss can be accommodated.

Nature has a seeming enjoyment of symmetry. We look symmetrical. We have two of most of everything. Scientists call this, 'bilaterally symmetric evolution', but it is misleading. We are almost completely asymmetrical. We have a dominant or preferred ear, eye, hand and so on. Try being blindfolded and then attempt to walk in a straight line for as long as possible. You may discover you have one leg longer than the other! The human brain appears to be the same left and right but it, too, is asymmetrical. It has developed this way for a purpose. Understanding the asymmetry of our brain hemispheres leads us towards some of the most useful concepts relating to the human brain and learning.

From the very beginnings of life the brain begins to develop a purposeful asymmetry in its circuitry. This leads to some specialization of function on each side of the brain. This 'relative lateralization' influences how the mind represents and makes sense of everyday experience.

If you had bumped into a hunter-gatherer half a million years ago, could you have had a conversation? Would he, she or its brain have been built the same way as yours? Corballis[127] suggested that the humans who lived over 2 million years ago may have had speech specialization in the left hemisphere but our modern flexible and rapid style of speech did not begin to develop until 150,000 to 200,000 years ago. This came about when tools began to be made and used as part of everyday life. The language necessary to share their production and use is largely 'generative' and this is a function of the left hemisphere. Modern hemispheric asymmetry, he argues, derives from this period.

Human asymmetries are evident from birth if not earlier. Within two days of being born, children given solutions of distilled water, sugar water and citric acid showed approach or withdrawal signals with activation in different hemispheres. There was an approach response to the sugar water and a withdrawal response to the citric acid. After tasting the sugar water there was consistently more activity in the left hemisphere. Approach responses are clearly marked from the earliest.

Growth spurts in the child's brain are also lateralized. Between the ages of four and six the left frontal lobes grow more rapidly than the right. Between the ages of eight and ten there is greater incremental growth in the right frontal lobes.[128] There is also growth within different areas of each hemisphere during this time. Children use primitive communication tools in babbling and in pointing, both of which are lateralized. The child is using different hemispheres for each function. At six months there is greater activation during speech in the left hemisphere and during music in the right. By 12 months the response has become more marked, with the left hemisphere clearly responding to names and the right to non-human sounds such as clicks.

Asymmetry in the child's brain is apparent for emotional responses by the age of ten months. The frontal lobes are more active in perceiving and producing emotional response than the parietal lobes. The left frontal lobe is more active than the right in responding to positive emotions. Ten month olds were sat on their mother's laps and watched an actress on video. The actress made facial expressions that went from happy to sad, happy to sad. The children were wired to electrodes that helped detect electrical changes in the brain. When watching happy actress there was activity in the left frontal lobe. When watching sad actress there was very little activity. In a follow-up experiment it was shown that infants use similarly differing areas of the brain for expressing happiness and sadness.

Does the left hand know what the right is doing?

The brain has a counter-clockwise torque! The human brain is twisted counter-clockwise with frontal right lobes larger than frontal left and at the rear of the brain the visual cortex is larger on the left than on the right.

Your brain is more likely to be asymmetrical if you are right handed rather than left handed. There is a division of labour between your two hands. When you write you see this in action. Which hand writes? Which hand holds the page? Research conducted by Guiard in 1987 proposed that the two hands work in what he called a kinematic chain with the non-dominant hand conducting movements that were slow and laboured – low temporal and spatial frequency – and the dominant hand movements that were quick and precise.[129] The left hemisphere controls movement on the right side of your body and the right hemisphere controls movement on the left side of your body. In early childhood, a time when only gross movements are available to the brain, movement areas in the right hemisphere are more fully developed than movement areas in the left. Does this mean that the right hemisphere becomes better at those slow, laboured movements and thus becomes dominant for them?

Handedness is notoriously sensitive to changes in measures. Change the measure and we change the statistics over who is right and non-right handed. Over time and across cultures it seems that mankind has a consistent pattern of right handedness, with the pattern settling around 94 or 95 per cent of the population. There are slightly more males who are left handed than females. Older people are more likely to write with the right hand and throw with the left. Left handers in the Western world seem more susceptible to certain types of illness: migraine, allergies, thyroid problems and those of the autoimmune system. Coren and Halpern suggested that they died younger but it is difficult to establish what part handedness alone might play in this even if the statistics are held to be true.[130]

In Korea less than 1 per cent of the population are left handed, while in the USA it is nearer to 13 per cent. It is difficult to disentangle cultural norms from the statistics but a pattern can nevertheless be inferred.

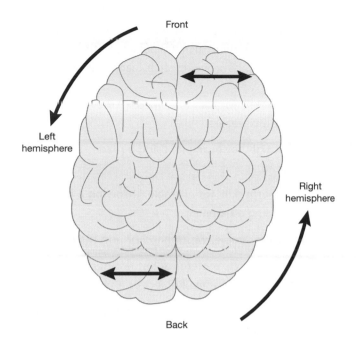

10.2 The brain develops through counter-clockwise torque and is larger on the right at the front and on the left at the back.

With left-handed writers there is no neurological evidence that inverted writers are wired differently from normal writers. Nor is there evidence that it arises because of some difference in motor control. The inverters who prefer the hooked position are about half of the left-handed population, though the figure goes down among the older generation and halves again if you are female. Research on inherited handedness is so contradictory it is not useful. There may be some basis for explaining handedness in the hormones your brain is awash with when you are in the womb.

After handedness, footedness is a good way of measuring hemispheric asymmetry. Which foot do you naturally kick the ball with? The warrior leads with the left foot and so do armies when marching. With right-handers over 90 per cent show a preference for the right foot when kicking but with left-handers it is very different. As a group, they do not seem as left footed as right-handers are right footed: 82 per cent of left-handers who preferred the left arm for throwing preferred the left foot for kicking; 78 per cent of left-handers who preferred the right arm for throwing preferred the right foot for kicking.

To collect information about handedness, questionnaires are often helpful. If you are only allowed one question, then it should be 'with which hand do you write?' If more, then here is how one research team classified the questions:

- Fine manual skill; for example, writing, drawing, holding a needle, using tweezers.

- Hand–wrist skill; for example, using a razor, combing hair, cutting bread.

- Hand–wrist–arm skill; for example, throwing a ball, holding a racquet, using a hammer.

- Strength; for example, which hand or arm is stronger.

- Activity that reflects preference but not necessarily skill; for example, picking up a small object or a book.

While we may have a preferred hand, foot, ear and eye, lateral preference for the eyes and the ears is less clearly expressed than hand preference. Watch people fold their arms and they will do so in a preferred way. Our body laterality expresses itself in the smallest of gestures: which eye do you wink with? Which hand claps and which is clapped? Oh and by the way, experiments with cats suggest that you cannot breed for paw preference. Does this mean that the teacher who is constantly changing the child's pen from the left to right hand is working against the 'grain' of the brain? Most probably.

A case has been made for identifying patterns of hemispheric dominance in a learner and linking those patterns to learning styles preference.[131] The evidence for this is less than substantial. First, it is difficult to assess hemispheric dominance meaningfully. Second, it is difficult to get clean evidence of hemispheric dominance without cultural or lifestyle influences. Third, the quantification of learning style preference itself is not secure: it is neither a science nor is it objective. This is an area where more work is required. There may be a way forward in looking at the prevalence of certain hormones in the brain. We do have evidence that bilateralism is associated with high mathematical ability (Benbow).[132] A high per cent of precocious children are left handed, mixed handed or have left-handed family. Why? Might it be to do with the levels of testosterone in the womb?

The left hemisphere is superior to the right for learning and using movements in sequence. This includes the sort of sucking and blowing in sequence that would be learned and used by playing a wind instrument. The right hemisphere is more useful in conveying the context of a series of gestures such as those used by a mime artist. These are not absolutes. Never allow yourself or anyone else in your hearing to say, 'I could have played like Courtney Pine but I'm too right brained!'

Language and hemisphericity

The left side of your brain is dominant for most language functions. This includes talking aloud, making sense of someone else speaking, picking up on sound changes, including changes of inflexion and voice tone and meanings of words. The right side is used for context. Damage to the right side of your brain might mean a difficulty in working out jokes, or innuendo, summarizing the gist of a passage of prose, reading satirical intent or understanding metaphor. Right hemisphere damage also leads to problems in decoding cartoons that have no language component.

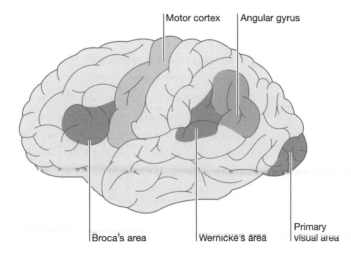

10.3 Different language functions reside in different parts of the brain predominating in the left hemisphere. In reading, the information is sent via the visual cortex and the angular gyrus to Wernicke's area. From here it is transferred from sensory data to motor impulses in Broca's area. Sounds are then structured together into language. Impairment of any stage leads to reading difficulties.

This is of significance in a formal learning environment such as a classroom. Often the language of the classroom is coded, ambiguous and negative: 'Now children, what do we not do when we go to assembly?' provokes certain complex decoding strategies. In work done with brain-damaged patients given similar indirect requests – 'can you play tennis?' – it was found that interpretation of the statement depended on where, in the brain, the damage had occurred. Ten subjects were asked to watch a film of such questions being asked.[133] Left-brain-damaged patients – Broca's aphasics – could easily decode the request and the appropriateness of the observed response. Right-brain-damaged patients could not. People with right-brain damage can understand the literal truth of a situation, but however, not always what it might mean in context. These patients were quite happy when, after being asked 'can you play tennis?', the match then took place in the front room.

A patient with hemispheric damage is told the first part of the joke we heard earlier:

> Patient: 'I've just swallowed a pillow.'
> Doctor: 'How do you feel?'

Then asked which of the following punchlines might be funniest,

> Patient: 'A little down in the mouth.'
> Patient: 'Full up.'
> Patient: 'Very sick. It's not easy to eat a pillow.'

would respond differently according to the hemisphere that was damaged. Those with damage to the right hemisphere might choose option three – 'Very sick. It's not easy to eat a pillow' – whereas a patient with damage to the left may choose option one. The patient with right-hemisphere damage chooses the one that offers literal truth.

The following facts apply to the lateralization of language in the brain:

 Language tends to be located in the left hemisphere for most humans.

 In a significant population of humans language occurs in both left and right hemispheres without any apparent loss of function.

▼ If an accident occurs and the left hemisphere is intact, speech production remains in the left hemisphere, speech comprehension migrates to the right even when the hemispheres are colossally disconnected.

▼ The left hemisphere suppresses the right hemisphere's speech potential.

▼ When the left hemisphere has been removed or badly damaged, the right hemisphere takes over language functions.

We do not know if there is a sensitive period for learning a second language. Nor do we know if the brain areas used for acquiring a second language are the same for different people. When we know answers to these questions we will be able to create the optimal conditions for language learning. Studies in bilingualism suggest that phonemes and grammar need to be learned young. Vocabulary and its meanings can be acquired throughout life. Is there such a thing as bilingualism? There is if you ask a citizen of the world. There is not if you ask a neuroscientist. Despite being able to move flawlessly between languages it is not the case that each of your languages has parity of status.

Scientists believe that one language is acquired in ways that make it the base or mother tongue. This is evident when we look at scans of the individual using that language and see activity in the left hemisphere. When the individual shifts to another language, different processing centres are involved. For this reason it is possible, not that it is recommended, to destroy the ability of a person to learn a new language by removing an area of the brain the size of your thumb. Language areas of the brain differ in subtle ways by individual and reflect that individual's history of language exposure. Using fMRI, Dr Joy Hirsch found that multilinguals used separate speech comprehension and speech production sites simultaneously. Wernicke's area – for comprehension – and Broca's area – for speech production – were activated separately. The exception was when the student had learned both languages in infancy. In which case, activation in Broca's area was the same for both languages. The competition for neural real estate makes it hard to learn a second language after puberty – the areas of the brain needed for the new language may have already been used for something else.[134]

Individuals with damage to the frontal lobes often tell tall tales. They 'confabulate' by telling stories that have no basis in truth without realizing they are doing so. There is no underlying psychopathology. No malice aforethought. It just happens.

Part of the explanation seems to lie, again, in the difference in function between left and right hemispheres. There is a higher incidence of confabulation among stroke patients. Stroke patients suffer localization of trauma and the brain seeks to compensate by having other parts of the brain take over the lost functions. This takes time and practice. Research done by Professor Ramachandran in San Diego explains confabulation as confused timing between left and right hemispheres.[135] Generally, the left hemisphere establishes the sense of the memory, while the right hemisphere detects anomalies or discrepancies in the experience. The left organizes the disparate chunks of experience and the right acts as interpreter. If there is damage to the right, as in some stroke cases, anomalies are no longer detected. The left hemisphere no longer has an interpreter to keep the experiences in check and confabulation takes place.

Deliberately stimulating the right hemisphere by squirting ice-cold water into the left ear of a confabulating patient temporarily relieved the confabulations. Professor Ramachandran believes that stimulating the right hemisphere, or inducing rapid eye movement (REM), through the sensory shock of the cold water temporarily evoked the retrieval of lost memories. When the water warmed the confabulations returned.

A favoured view is that in learning the left side is specialized for language and the right for spatial awareness. Another is that the left is better at focused attention tasks and that the right for more divergent or diffuse attention tasks. Yet another is that the left is analytic, while the right is holistic. The difficulty, posed by each of these dichotomies, is that there is a smattering of truth in each. However, no more than that. Accumulated research now suggests that we are unlikely to get a one-size-fits-all explanation of right and left difference. Both sides have involvement with most activity.

The right hemisphere does not always assess the holistic aspects of an object more effectively than the left hemisphere, nor does the left hemisphere

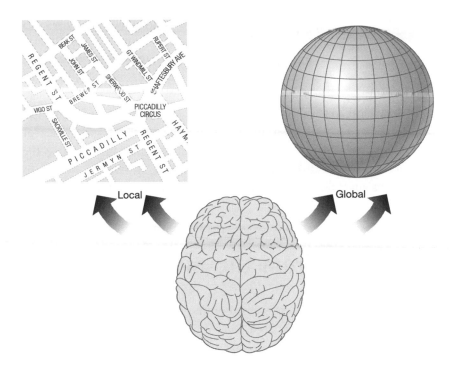

10.4 Left and right hemispheres differ in the way they process information, not in their structures.

always assess finer details more effectively than the right hemisphere.[136] It is believed that the left hemisphere is better at processing visual–spatial information of high frequency and the right at processing visual–spatial information of low frequency. The hemispheres differ in the way they process and not in their structures. When we look at an object, some scientists believe that the left hemisphere makes more use of a categorization system that gives good information about the relative position of the object, while the right simultaneously uses a co-ordinate system giving information about distance and specific location. The hemispheres form a single integrated information processing system but they allocate attention differently. Need dictates the processing system and thus the hemisphere that gets used.

The corpus callosum is the major fibre tract connecting the two hemispheres. It has at least 200 million nerve fibres and acts like a conduit relaying some sorts of information left and right. There is considerable variation in the size of the corpus callosum by gender and by handedness. Left-handers have larger areas of the corpus callosum. This is more pronounced if you are left handed and male. Females generally have a larger corpus callosum. There is little evidence that a larger corpus callosum improves hemispheric integration. Those who argue that women's seemingly better ability to multi-task, to communicate under stress and to be 'intuitive' must look elsewhere for a biological explanation. The corpus callosum also functions as an inhibitory barrier. Activation in one hemisphere inhibits the level of excitation in the other. The corpus callosum plays a part in regulating the level of activation between the two hemispheres. It also contributes to reducing maladaptive cross-talk between the two halves of the brain.

Stay away from the medicine man

So much of classroom success is based on the management of emotions. So much of emotion is, and has been, shaped by attention. Your brain cannot possibly process all the sensory information it receives so it gives some stimuli attention and others it neglects. The technical terms are 'attended' and 'unattended' stimuli. It is there and you notice it, or it is there but it is ignored on your behalf.

What is attended or unattended depends on goals and needs, which are in turn shaped by, among other things, experience and what you have done with it. When you decide you have had enough attending, you discontinue and this is known as extinction or habituation. This is the 'done that got the T-shirt of human attentional systems'. When your attention is engaged this is known as 'vigilance'. Vigilance is the equivalent of the 'watch out for the timeshare salesman' of human attentional systems. The evidence suggests that the systems that run attention are asymmetrically organized in the brain.

Patients with damage to the right hemisphere have poorer levels of sustained attention than patients with similar left-hemisphere damage. It seems the right hemisphere is more active during a sustained attention task than the left. The right hemisphere also plays a dominant role in controlling arousal and shows more sensitivity to pain than the left. Patients with right-brain damage showed higher pain endurance than those with left-brain damage.

Emotions such as sadness or joy are run by separate systems in the brain. Increased activity on the right side of the brain can be a signal of depression. Increased activity on the left can signal happiness, even euphoria.

Work done at the University of Wisconsin shows how people with more chemical and electrical activity in the left hemisphere have a more positive all-round mood, while people with more chemical and electrical activity in the right hemisphere have a more negative all-round mood.[137] Some drugs are more effective on one side of the brain than the other: drugs that depend on dopamine are more effective in the left hemisphere; drugs that depend on norepinephrine are more effective in the right hemisphere.

Researchers at Johns Hopkins University have identified an area of the brain that appears to be activated when we dwell on negative personal experiences. Subjects asked to describe family crises, financial worries and situations of personal stress on tape and then listen to the tapes showed more PET scan activity in the right frontal lobe as they did so. The right frontal lobe contributes to goal-setting, planning and evaluation of

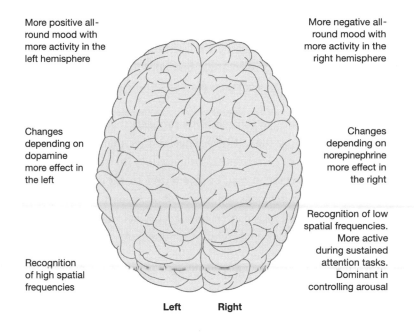

More positive all-round mood with more activity in the left hemisphere

More negative all-round mood with more activity in the right hemisphere

Changes depending on dopamine more effect in the left

Changes depending on norepinephrine more effect in the right

Recognition of low spatial frequencies. More active during sustained attention tasks. Dominant in controlling arousal

Recognition of high spatial frequencies

Left   **Right**

10.5 The systems that run attention are asymmetrically organized in the brain.

decisions. When the same subjects were asked to listen to tapes of themselves describing inconsequential everyday events there was correspondingly less activity in the right frontal lobe. The Johns Hopkins' staff infer that some of the neural structures to do with 'worry' lie in the right frontal lobe. All of which is very worrying.

Type 'A' personalities are more coronary prone. The type 'A' personality is most often a man and one who exhibits hostility, anger and impatience. The way the brain mediates emotion may play a part in exposing some of us to early death through heart attacks. Work with animals shows that anger induction can induce myocardial ischaemia. Depressives are also more susceptible to sudden cardiac arrest.

In 1942 a classic study of voodoo death showed that tribesmen died within hours of being cursed by a medicine man.[138] Studies with animals show that emotional stress can reduce the threshold for ventricular fibrillation. It can give you a heart attack. Brain mechanisms regulating emotion can play a significant part in inducing sudden death. A very good friend of mine had a family member who, after a lifetime of working in the local mill in a management position, was told that his services were no longer required. Due to a decline in business he and others were being made redundant. It was Friday morning. That afternoon he died at home of a heart attack. Of the 300,000 deaths through cardiac arrest annually in the USA, it is estimated that in 20 per cent of cases emotion plays a significant role.

The brain heart laterality hypothesis (BHL) suggests that the degree to which emotion is regulated by the left hemisphere rather than the norm, which is the right hemisphere, correlates to vulnerability to sudden death. In an explanation of why emotion may be lateralized to the right hemisphere of your brain, Lane and Jennings argue that it is in part to do with natural selection.[139] Natural selection confers greater survival value on those who can maximize cardiac output in survival situations. At the same time brain asymmetry conferred greater cognitive abilities. What natural selection did not anticipate was the impact of diseases associated with unrelieved stress or with elongated survival – most sudden heart attack deaths occur in middle age – and so we have a brain that is lateralized for both emotional and intellectual demands. In circumstances when the lateralization is irregular, you are correspondingly more vulnerable to unforeseen change.

The eyes have it

Work on seeing and hearing shows that we process the information we see or hear with different sides of the brain according to the source of information. In seeing everyday objects the information that comes to our eyes is split up before being sent to the left or the right side of the brain. When I stare at an object, the right side of my brain processes information seen by the right side of both retinas. The left side processes information seen by the left side of both retinas. A mechanism known as the optic chasm is the crossing point for this information. The left field of an object I am staring at is seen by the right side of each retina and the right field by the left side of each retina. Patients with split brains have difficulty perceiving whole objects that they are seeing. They can 'see' the object but have difficulty making it whole. If the corpus callosum is cut and the eyes and the head are kept still, each hemisphere can only see half of what is in front of it.

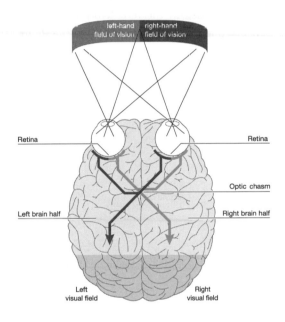

10.6 The optic pathways provide a cross-over of information via the optic chasm.

The visual system is based on simultaneous aggregating and dis-aggregating. As we see everyday objects the information is broken down and then sent simultaneously to separate halves of the brain where it is reassembled albeit in different but entirely complementary ways.

The notion of 'simultaneous aggregating and dis-aggregating' is useful in thinking about the learning brain. In a learning challenge the process is constant. The learner switches from the detail to the Big Picture, back and forth, back and forth. When Big Picture information is missing, switching becomes slower, more messy and dislocated. Learning needs us to be able to locate the detail in the wider context. The structure and organization of the brain points us to this basic learning premise: seek and secure connections and constantly locate those connections in the wider context.

The Japanese language has a phonetic system known as Kana and a pictographic system known as Kanji. In research conducted with normal subjects in both systems nonsense words were shown in the right and left field of vision and a difference was found. The sound system of Kana tends to be processed in the left hemisphere, while the visual system of Kanji is processed in the right.[140] In his book *The Right Mind* (1997), Robert Ornstein points out that 'Japanese people who suffer brain lesions in the left temporal hemisphere lose their ability to process phonetic Kana, both in reading and writing, but can still process logographic Kanji; whereas those suffering lesions in the left parietoccipital area suffer impaired processing of Kanji but not Kana.'

MEANING	KANA	KANJI
INK	インキ (INKI)	墨 (KANJI)
UNIVERSITY	ダイガク (DAIGAKU)	大学 (GREAT LEARNING)
TOKYO	トウキヨウ (TOKYO)	東京 (EAST CAPITAL)

10.7 In Japan there are two forms of writing: Kana is syllabic; Kanji is ideographic.

The right hemisphere is more sensitive to low spatial frequencies and the left to high, thus faces or letters may be processed more effectively by one or the other dependent on their spatial frequency characteristics. However, the consensus is that this becomes more dynamic with different types of processing. With early perceptual stages of processing there is right hemisphere advantage and at later cognitive levels there is left hemisphere advantage.

Listen to me when I'm talking

We are dichotic listeners! This means you listen differently by ear. In some telephone sales techniques courses participants are asked to switch the phone from ear to ear depending on the purpose of the call. If you are wishing to close that sale and be matter of fact, attentive to detail and focused on figures, then switch to your right ear. If you wish to be warm and empathetic in your listening, engage with the emotional tone of the conversation and are in no hurry, then switch to the left.

What you hear in your right ear is processed by the language centres in the left hemisphere. Information is passed simultaneously to both left and right hemispheres but it is in the left hemisphere that language processing predominates. When experiments were conducted with subjects listening in one ear, different information could still be processed in the other ear to a certain degree. Dichotic listening tasks (DL) are used to assess laterality, particularly in language processing. There appears to be what is known as Right Ear Advantage (REA). With dichotic listening, normal subjects report words presented to the right ear more accurately than to the left. Meaningless vowel symbols and words played backwards also demonstrate left hemisphere/right ear advantage. Some non-verbal sounds such as bird song, the melodic component of a musical piece, a dog barking, a ship's siren show advantage in the right hemisphere.

Research completed in the 1960s and 1970s found that children showed better recall from the right compared with the left ear with one set of stimulus sounds. Morton and Kershner found that normal-achieving children achieved differently from children with reading difficulties on a DL task when tested in the morning but not in the afternoon.[141] The normal-achieving children were more strongly lateralized compared to the reading difficulties children when instructed to listen selectively to the right ear input as opposed to either or to the sounds in their left ear. This may indicate a lack of attentional resources in the morning for children with reading difficulties.

What does this mean for the telephone sales force? There is probably more value in the belief that switching makes a difference than in any subtle difference offered by dichotic listening. Like many of the myths around left and right brain this one has a tiny grain of truth.

So what can we conclude about left and right?

The differences in function are relative and not absolute. The left brain is not only involved in motor control and higher order functioning but also seems to be important in the autoimmune system. The right brain is more involved in the control of vital functions involving survival, coping with stress and with external challenges. There are more chemicals to do with emotional arousal and inhibition in the right hemisphere.

Scientific understanding has until very recently relied on post mortem study of dysfunction – including split-brain patients – or invasive techniques to find out about the workings of the brain. Nowadays blood and oxygen changes can be measured, overlaid with MRI and mapped and we can see the tremendous individual variance between left and right. Cerebral dominance is still a widely used term by specialists in this field. Researchers are more concerned with the degrees of, rather than absolute, difference between left and right. They are more likely to be considering differences between the top and the bottom, the front and the back of each hemisphere.

Facts about the left and right hemispheres of the brain:

They are not identical in their capability or their organization.

They are both involved in all complex tasks.

They differ significantly in how language is understood and produced.

They process complex spatial relationships differently.

The neurotransmitters that regulate attention, motor behaviour approach-withdrawal and self-regulation differ in their distribution.

Male and female brains differ in their asymmetry, which is largely due to hormonal levels within the womb.

There is little evidence to suggest that either one or the other hemisphere turns on to perform a specific task all by itself – there are many areas of the brain involved in the simplest of tasks.

What might this mean for formal learning?

Much learning is curiosity driven but you do not 'do' curiosity. It is not timetabled for a double period on Friday afternoon, nor is it on page 43 of the workbook. Damage to the hippocampus leads to lack of curiosity. Curiosity directs attention. Attention is at the core of cognitive engagement.

The idea of 'whole-brain' learning has more metaphorical than scientific value. Too restricted a diet stunts growth. Too much of the same leads to boredom. If you want to grow plants to a particular shape, confine their space. There is no such thing as a right- or a left-brain learner but there are such things as stultifying learning environments, a slavish attachment to monotony and restricted thinking about what is and is not good learning.

There is nothing in the research of hemispheric difference that says teach like this or else. If you look closely at what it tells us, it tells us to respect individuality and to engage the attentional systems. To this end I think the following common-sense learning approaches are consistent with some of the research outcomes into asymmetry. The list is not prescriptive. Nor is it surprising that it reads like what the best classroom teachers have been instinctively doing for years.

Multiple level engagement

Assume multiple entry and exit points in the design of learning. This cannot be done if all learners are expected to do the same thing, for the same duration, with the same success measures.

Global and local emphasis

When designing learning activities or inputs of new information be aware of the need to provide a global context within which local data can sit.

Aggregate and dis-aggregate

Secure opportunities for learners to build up and break down. Make it a regular part of their learning. If, for example, you are teaching a Shakespearian sonnet, it makes sense to look at what the author wants to evoke in the reader as well as the techniques he uses to achieve that response. Alternatively start with the smallest unit, the sound, and build up.

Sort by similarity and retrieve by difference

Teaching classification skills, practising identifying and specifying similarity and difference, generating comparative data and organizational models are all ways of developing sort and retrieve capability.

Seek connections

At all levels and at all times, meaningful learning involves seeking and securing connections. An accomplished learner is practised in surveying material for connections. An accomplished educator builds this into everyday classroom interactions.

Cross-lateral learning

Impose an occasional regime where a deliberate mix of visual and auditory learning co-exists. For example, a learner self-consciously describes aloud what he is thinking as he constructs a graph or diagram.

Mimicry and gesture

Using open and closed movements – excitatory and inhibitory – learners practise through gesture. If you are able to mimic chemical transmission at the synapse and do so successfully, then learning has begun.

Learning materials

Design learning materials to allow easy 'switching' from high to low visual frequency and vice versa. At the simplest level this could mean larger and more open fonts in poster form for summary information alongside body text. Position these summary visuals in the left field.

Bilateral classrooms

Check for lateralization using some of the measures described above. Allow learners to find the hand they are comfortable writing with. Have left-handed equipment – for example, scissors – as standard in every classroom.

Sight and hearing lines

Where do teachers position themselves when giving information or asking questions? Does the teacher's physical position ensure she can be easily seen and heard? Use a recognized space on the classroom floor to 'hit the spot'. Use it when giving vital summary information. Observe how children cock their heads to hear. Which ear predominates? Rotate their physical position from time to time

In the next chapter we consider another possible dimension of difference: male and female brains.

Chapter 11

Gender:

how do we respect difference?

This chapter contains the following sections:

⚔ **Starting early**
Differences in male and female brains exist but are not absolute. Are there degrees of male or femaleness evident in a brain? Might there be sites within the brain that are more male or female? When do differences emerge?

⚔ **Let's not jump to conclusions!**
There is little basis in science for teaching boys and girls in different ways. The dangers of mis-interpretation.

⚔ **Do boys and girls learn differently?**
Practical case studies that explore possible differences.

⚔ **What are the differences?**
What research describes as the difference in learning behaviours of men and women.

⚔ **Can't we just talk about it?**
Differences in language functions between men and women.

⚔ **Mathematical reasoning**
Boys and girls approach mathematics in different ways. Why?

⚔ **Your motor movement's gross!**
Manipulating yourself or an object through space. Significant differences in the way men and women do this. The gestures right- and left-handers make.

... and will answer the following questions:

- ▷ At what point does a brain begin to be recognizably male or female?

- ▷ Should we teach boys and girls separately?

- ▷ Do boys and girls learn differently?

- ▷ What are the major differences in the learning behaviours of men and women?

- ▷ Are women better designed for language?

- ▷ What sorts of things should I do when teaching maths to make it boy/girl friendly?

- ▷ Who is more likely to be better at multi-tasking: men or women?

Introduction

One evening a woman found her partner standing over their baby's crib. Silently she watched him. As he stared down at the sleeping infant, she saw the look of awe and wonder on his face. She sensed an engagement and curiosity she had never noticed in him before. His face was a mixture of emotions: tenderness, doubt and delight, amazement and mystification. She slipped her arm around his. 'A penny for your thoughts,' she said. 'It's amazing!' he replied. 'I just don't see how anyone can make a crib like that for £29.95.'

Males and females behave differently. They look different. Their bodies are different. Do they learn differently? Some popular writers claim there are differences in male and female brains. If so, what are the differences? How significant are they? How do differences in the architecture of male and female brains map onto differences in how we think, remember and learn? In what ways might such differences be a reflection of evolutionary history or of differing roles in society or of the way society and science tends to look for and position such differences? Might such differences play any part in learning preference?

Starting early

Female brains are less lateralized. Males show a greater lateralization of function. There are differences in the asymmetry of male and female brains. Hormonal levels within the womb contribute significantly to the extent of the difference.

By the age of six months, research[142] shows that the girls' left hemisphere is developing faster than their right, while the opposite is true for boys. These gender differences have been linked with hormonal differences. Testosterone improves spatial memory and increases hippocampus size in male and female birds. At different times of the year, when navigation is important for finding and storing food, for example, the hippocampus grows. The hippocampus is essential in visual and spatial recall. In an investigation of spatial abilities in women during their monthly hormonal cycles, it was found that women's spatial ability was inversely related to their levels of oestrogen.[143] This has implications for taking exams. If a girl is studying an academic subject that requires insight into the organization of shapes, spatial relationships, objects rotated in space or unfolded, then sitting an exam when your oestrogen levels are awry could lead to difficulties.

Testosterone is largely responsible for gender differences in asymmetry in the brain. Every organism requires multiple levels of control over maleness and femaleness. It is a fascinating thought to recognize the number of areas of the brain in which gender differences exist, each with its own development timetable, its own mode of responding to hormonal levels, its own mechanisms for interacting with other parts of the brain. It is as if we are saying that different parts of your brain are more male or female than other parts – you have a very female emotional circuitry but are very male in your perceptual systems; I have a very female memory system but my musculature is very male.

In the central nervous system alone, the differentiation of sexual behaviours involves sexual dimorphism of the hypothalamus, preoptic area, amygdala, pituitary, spinal cord nuclei associated with pelvic musculature, perhaps the cortex, perhaps the hippocampus, perhaps the pineal body; gender differences in exploratory behaviour may involve cerebral cortex, striatum and hippocampus; gender differences in paternal and maternal behaviour involve the hypothalamus, pituitary, and probably additional brain regions as well; gender differences in perception involve differential organization of a variety of sensory processing pathways and associative connections.[144]

Let's not jump to conclusions!

Before we look at what science has got to tell us about the learning of men and women, boys and girls, we shall start with a few caveats.[145]

 Variability within the sexes is as significant as variability between the sexes. There is a great deal of overlap in the distribution of ability across men and women.

▼ Despite research on differences in male and female brains demonstrating clear differences, the results are too often equivocal and subject to different interpretation. It is difficult to get 'clean' outcomes.

▼ Gender differences in higher mental functions are typically on the order of one-fourth of a standard deviation.

▼ Premature articulation of findings. Because some rats happened to navigate successfully through a maze and, they happened to be male, it does not mean women cannot read maps!

▼ Gender remains no better a determinant for shaping educational policy than handedness, limb length or shoe size.

The real danger is in the possible misuse of emerging findings about male and female brains. What we do not want is whimsy trickling into educational policy. While there may be practical or religious reasons for strategies such as single-sex schooling, or separating boys and girls in science, or sitting in boy–girl pairings, there is nothing in brain science that says *do this!*

Science has demonstrated some clear physical differences between male and female brains. Male brains, although larger and heavier, are – surprisingly for some – less dense. A team from McMaster University, Ontario, Canada found that women's brains are more tightly packed with cells in the frontal lobe.[146] This is an area that controls mental processes such as judgement, personality, planning and working memory. They found that women have up to 15 per cent more brain cell density, which controls the so-called higher mental processes. However, as they get older, women appear to shed cells more rapidly from this area than men. By middle age, the density is similar for both sexes.

Here we have in cameo the problem for researchers. What conclusions should be drawn? Could we infer from this that women naturally have better judgement, more personality, more astute planning and remember where they put things? I will leave that to you. Greater density of cells does not mean that women can out-perform men. It could be one way by which nature ensures that women can perform adequately despite the smaller size of their brain.

Male brains are larger in the anterior temporal lobes, an area that is just in front of the ears. This area includes the amygdala, an area associated with emotional arousal, and the anterior hippocampus, which is associated with long-term memory. A major study also found that the anterior cingulate cortex, another area involved in emotional sensitivity, is larger in women.[147] In face-processing tasks gifted males had significantly inhibited left hemisphere activity. The suggestion is that this specialization allowed less interference for the right hemisphere to check for affective context. Female subjects were bilaterally engaged during face processing.

The corpus callosum is larger in women and this is independent of handedness and there is a tendency towards larger absolute callosal areas in women. Some writers have seized on this as evidence of women being better at communicating when under stress, multi-tasking and intuitive insight. They argue that the corpus callosum provides a more efficient relay system for whole-brain integration. It is better at 'whole-brain functioning', therefore the woman ought also to be better at holistic behaviours. The science behind this is weak. In general the neuroscience of gender is fascinating and sometimes conflicting. It points to a correlation between hemispheric organization and gender differences, but it is difficult to route this through to specific behavioural patterns.

The consequences of brain injury differ between male and females. In some studies damage to the left hemisphere of male brains resulted in impaired verbal IQ more than non-verbal IQ with damage to right hemisphere showing lowered non-verbal performance compared to verbal. Women showed no effect of side of lesion. Language and spatial abilities are more bilaterally controlled in females than in males.

Nature and nurture explanations can be made. Ontogeny reflects phylogeny. The organization of your brain reflects its interactions with its environment. If you constantly interact with the world around you in patterned ways, and all of your forebears who have provided you with your genetic structure have done the same, then who is able to say if your brain has shaped, or is shaped by, those interactions? Are the differences innate or have they been learned?

Despite accumulated evidence from cognitive psychologists that men and women perform in tests in very different ways, it is a bold leap to say that they are so different we should teach them in different ways. Perhaps science will eventually provide some answers?

Do boys and girls learn differently?

In a BBC television programme called *Women on Top* we began to test some of the differences. I collaborated with a London school and Professor John Williams, a mathematician who works for MENSA (the UK organization for people of high intelligence), to devise tests on behalf of the BBC. To start we set out to examine some physical differences.

Are there swerving differences? Males and females demonstrate propensities to turn either left or right. It is affected by dopamine. Females turn more. Females turn more to the left. In a test that was simply used as a means of identifying locomotory differences we asked six year olds to run through a set of cones positioned in a play area at about a metre apart. This swerve test involved four boys and four girls. We asked them to run it again and again. What we noticed was, at this age, the boys tended to be better at moving independently off either foot, they used their arms more and they were more competitive. The boys have physical advantages that make this task easier. They seemed to be better at manipulating themselves in two dimensions. Might they also be better at manipulating objects in two or three dimensions?

Are there play differences? We then observed boys and girls in the play area at morning break and at lunch. We recorded some of what happened on film. These were children between the ages of five and ten. While the many individual differences were obvious, some patterns of children's play emerged.

As we observed, the boys seemed to command more of the physical space of the play area. They ran around more. There was more exploration of the perimeter by boys. They interacted in smaller social groupings. They appeared to be more competitive but less focused in their play. Games were more fluid, beginning and ending haphazardly and with changing participation. We tried to identify isolates. Boys seemed to remain on their own for longer. As a general rule, girls played with girls and boys with boys. This pattern broke down in one-off interactions between an individual boy and girl from time to time, but the tendency was for separate play.

The girls seemed less robust in their use of physical play. They ran around less and confined their physical play to more limited areas of the playground. An interesting cameo was observed in morning break. A group of five girls brought out some toys such as wobble boards, hoops and skipping ropes. They began to use these toys to play individually. Very quickly a group of boys commandeered the wobble boards, hoops and skipping ropes and took them off for their own use. Shortly after, the girls got them back again when the boys abandoned them for some new activity!

We observed a higher proportion of girls on the periphery of the main play area. Many sat against, by, or on top of a wall. They did so in social groups. Mostly small units of three or four, but in one case a large group of girls sat side by side on a wall observing proceedings and engaged in conversation. The girls who played in groups out in the play area were focused by the activity or by the prop. We observed skipping to what appeared to be rules. We also observed turn taking using hoops.

Are there differences in throwing? We replicated a test conducted by Kimura and Lunn involving throwing a velcro covered ball underhand towards a horizontal target. We repeated the test overhand. This was done with five year olds, the original test investigated boys' and girls' abilities in targeting between the ages of three and five. Boys were significantly better in the former and dramatically better in the latter.

Might different phases of physical development and experience of targeting activities in sport account for the difference? Undoubtedly, but as they get older the differences may well remain. Men would appear to be better at accurate throwing and catching than women. One of the most widely recognized differences between men and women is in throwing objects at a target. Factors such as muscle tone and bulk, bone density and length, endurance, strength and speed may also contribute to the differences.

Men may also gain more satisfaction from the completion of an activity in which they are more likely to succeed than their female peers. They may thus be more likely to practise and reinforce success. There may also be real differences that persist over and above temporary variables.

In research involving men and women throwing darts, the men were more consistently accurate than the women by at least a full standard deviation. In a similar experiment conducted in the same lab, men were better at an interception task.[148] What is interesting about this work is that there was no correlation between performance in tasks that might be thought to demand similar abilities such as mental rehearsals of spatial information. This suggests that targeting is a 'relatively separate ability'.

The tests we ran attempted first to establish certain, obvious, differences in the physical dispositions of the boys and girls. Having done this, we then ran tests to look at cognitive differences.

These test were conducted with pupils from Year 1 of Horsenden Primary School in Ealing, London. Tania Borsig, the class teacher, is of the view that the boys and girls in her class 'behave differently and learn differently, but don't achieve differently'. We set out to research some of her observed patterns of behaviour.

Are there differences in simple construction tasks? We were interested if offered the choice of Scrabble or Lego, would the boys choose Lego and the girls Scrabble? As in all great research traditions, we started with a setback. There was not a strong pattern of preference based on gender across the class. Secretly, I was pleased. We then moved to an activity that had more 'science' behind it – a test of reaction to concrete apparatus. What strategies are used when boys and girls are given multi-coloured, multi-shaped slabs to 'sort'?

In single-sex friendship pairs, and separately, with minimal prompting, the boys and girls were asked to play with the plastic blocks. What happened again and again was that the boys sorted by function and the girls by some classificatory system. The girls built low, flat and extended connected structures. The boys went high and independent. The boys' structures threatened to topple. The girls' structures threatened to fall off the edge of the table. When asked, what they had produced, the boys cited phenomena from the outside world: Pokémon characters, a castle, a car. The girls used words like 'shapes', 'pictures', 'tessellations'. The boys experimented a little more and seemed willing to start again. The girls settled into a pattern of performance. There was less observed collaboration with the boys. The girls occasionally found each other a suitable colour or shape. Throughout all the experiments the BBC television cameras rolled.

And therein is the key to this. The experiments were done because of their visual quality. They were also done because they would lend something to a television programme whose thesis was: if the brains of boys and girls are so different, ought we to be teaching them in different ways? We set up one final experiment to further test the thesis.

Are there differences in switching from a routine? We organized boys and girls in three teams of three: nine boys, nine girls. The children were ten years old and randomly selected. The test they were to do was a variation on the Luchins water jar test. The original test involved problems of the kind, 'You have a 4-pint jar, a 5-pint jar and a 7-pint jar. Using as few pourings as possible how do you measure out 2 pints of water?'

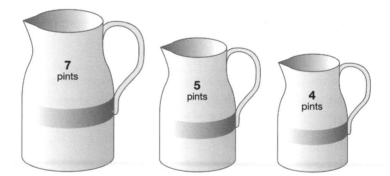

11.1 With water jugs of different capacity can you pour the water between the jugs so as to be left with two units? How long will it take? What will be your method?

Traditionally, the subjects are shown how to solve the problem using all three jars, then do a few problems requiring three jars, then encounter a problem admitting either three or two jars, then one requiring two jars. They tend not to notice the opportunity to use two jars in the penultimate problem or to be able to see how to do so when required in the final problem. These two test problems can be introduced earlier in the series and the subjects still resist switching to the simpler solution. Previous research suggests that girls develop a habitual approach to solution earlier in the series than boys do and are less likely to switch.

What happened in practice was the reverse! Perhaps our sample was not large enough? Perhaps we had not been sufficiently rigorous in setting up the conditions? Maybe we did not run it enough times? Or perhaps we had just got a reminder that life and learning is a lot messier than theorists would sometimes like. The girls were no less adept at switching than the boys.

Both sets of three followed similar paths of hypothesizing, mini-trials, debating and speculating then agreeing to get on with it. We had expected the girls to become accomplished very quickly, to fall into a pattern and be more resistant to breaking out of that pattern. We had also expected that they would be able to accommodate other simultaneous challenges, provided they did not have to break out of the pattern. We thought they might be quicker to habituate. As it happened there was considerable ingenuity and flexibility among both boys and girls. One outcome that did conform to our expectations was that under stress, the boys' performance lifted disproportionately to the girls. Against the challenge of getting a result in a limited time they did much better.

It is against the context of these limited but useful experiments that we can examine what cognitive scientists say about the differences between men and women.

What are the differences?

The lists opposite are compiled from a variety of published sources that look at behavioural differences. They do not have their immediate origin in brain research. We cannot with any authority surmise that they are prevalent as a result of architectural differences in male and female brains. This would be a 'bridge too far'. They do, however, pose questions that, at some time in the future, neuroscientists may like to try and answer: **Why is it that ... ?**

Women do better on:

- tasks that involve perceptual speed such as the ability to rapidly identify matching items.

- most language functions.

- tasks of ideational fluency (for example, list objects of the same colour) and on verbal fluency (for example, words that begin with the same letter).

- tasks that involve arithmetic calculation.

- remembering whether an object or a series of objects has been displaced.

- controlling distal musculature – muscles further from the trunk.

- precise manual control such as replicating finger-tip touching patterns.

- co-ordinating several movements together.

- rapid access and retrieval of information from memory.

- landmark as opposed to geometrical navigation.

- remembering faces and associating them with feelings.

- studying by separating things out, practising until successful then moving on to the next.

Men do better on:

- tasks that are spatial in nature, such as navigation in two and three dimensions, and maze performance.

- mechanical skills including assembling pictures, manipulating blocks and mental rotation of objects.

- ⚡ guiding or intercepting projectiles using gross motor movement.

- ⚡ simple repetitive movements such as hitting a single key.

- ⚡ tasks that involve mathematical calculation.

- ⚡ seeing and thinking in concepts and patterns, finding abstract relationships and forming links between them.

- ⚡ concentrating on an abstract idea or theorem and dissociating it from other 'distracting' information.

- ⚡ disembedding shapes from surroundings.

- ⚡ covert counting (in their heads).

- ⚡ persisting longer in covert retrieval (answering from memory).

- ⚡ geometrical as opposed to landmark navigation.

- ⚡ atomizing a task and therefore persisting with it (mature males).

Can't we just talk about it?

There appears to be a gender difference in those areas of the brain contributing to speech and language, although the findings are intriguing rather than definitive. In processing of speech sounds, brain activation in males is triggered to the left inferior frontal gyrus, whereas the pattern in females is for more diffuse neural systems involving both hemispheres.

An area crucial for language comprehension in the left temporal lobe, the planum temporale, is more highly activated during language tasks in males than in women. A listening study of 20 men and 20 women found men use the left side of the brain – traditionally associated with understanding language – to pick up conversations. But women also used the right side. Participants listened to excerpts from John Grisham's novel *The Partner* while the researchers from Indiana University School of Medicine monitored reactions using fMRI.[149] Scientists have considered that male brains are more lateralized than female brains for some time. One view is that language centres are more tightly located in male brains and more widely dispersed in female brains.

Consider this task. In your head, go through the alphabet and count the number of letters that end in the sound 'ee'. Including 'e', how many are there? Now go through the alphabet again, and this time count how many capital letters there are that have curves. Do it in your head. How many are there?

Your score may reflect your gender: females, on average, tend to do better on the sound task; males, on average, tend to do better on the shape task.[150]

Females, on average, perform better than males in skills that require the use of language. These include verbal fluency, speed of articulation and grammar. In word tasks gifted subjects activated the frontal regions of the brain to a greater extent than control subjects who tended to activate temporal regions. Girls in the West tend to speak earlier than boys. Their vocabulary is larger earlier. Statistics quoted light-heartedly by memory researcher Marilee Springer suggest that women in the West use about 7,000 words on average daily and men about 2,000. Which leaves the question: what do you do when you are with a man and his quota is met? However, parents in the West contribute to the phenomenon by talking differently to their sons and daughters and by having different expectations around behaviour and about social interaction and play. If you are a parent, audit the way you talk to your sons and daughters for a day. Look at the distribution of praise and sanction. Who gets it and for what? By implication, this balance of praise and sanction, the noticing that goes with it, reinforces certain patterns of behaviour. You get more of what you reinforce. This leads to the heart of the issue. When was the last time your daughter was praised for risk taking and physical prowess, for persistence, scoring high on the computer game, for 'being like daddy'? When was the last time your son was praised for tidiness, neatness, accuracy in schoolwork, reading a story to its end, playing quietly, sharing toys, saying something correctly, 'helping mummy'?

Mathematical reasoning

An OECD report published in December 2001 reported a worldwide disparity between the reading literacy of boys and girls.[151] At present, boys are performing poorer than girls in reading the world over. OECD also reported that worldwide there was no such disparity in maths and in many countries boys were slightly ahead. When interviewed by the ASCD for its journal *Educational Leadership*, Brian Butterworth explained that women were far more likely to self-denigrate their abilities in maths and undervalued their performance.[152] In the UK his research shows no difference on average in the public examination performance of boys and girls.

According to MENSA, boys are more likely to be highly talented in mathematics than girls.[153] Girls are better on calculations and males better on mathematical reasoning. Work done on spatial tasks shows that on average men outperform women in tasks that are spatial in nature, including maze performance, picture assembly, block design, mental rotation, and certain mechanical skills. They are also more adept at disembedding shapes from their surroundings.

Carr and Jessup[154] observed that boys and girls engage different processes for everyday calculations. Girls use procedural, overt counting such as touching their fingers better and more often to find their answers than boys. Boys were more successful with covert counting such as in their heads. Boys persisted longer in trying to retrieve from memory though they were worse at it than girls, who used other backup strategies. Girls are more likely to see each area of study as an entity and need to feel confident about it before they can then move on to the next. The boys are more likely to be 'atomizers'. They can dissociate the task at hand more readily. They get better at persisting as they get older, particularly if they have atomized a task. Testosterone may play a part in resisting fatigue to allow this to occur.

Boys are more likely to see and think in concepts and patterns, finding abstract relationships and forming links between them. Mature males find it easier to concentrate on an abstract idea or theorem and dissociate it from other 'distracting' information.

Here are some ideas to help both boys and girls develop all-round mathematical ability:

 Use lots of physical objects that boys and girls can get their hands on, feel, unfold and relate to the two-dimensional version in their workbook.

 In class use number fans, whiteboards and paired pre-discussion to ensure that processing time occurs before answers are volunteered. Thoughtful answers are always better than quick answers.

 Provide opportunities for individuals to talk through their thinking as the experience occurs.

 Use the descriptive, reflective, speculative discipline: 'this is what I notice', 'I think it happens because', 'the next time I do it I will ...'

 Break down tasks into the smallest unit, review for understanding and consolidation before moving on.

 Reward for persistence and risk taking and not just neatness and accuracy.

 Connect to life. Avoid rote homework and replace with shorter, real-life application homework, which does not need teacher marking because it is discussed extensively in class.

Your motor movement's gross!

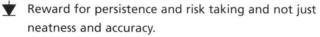

The right side of your brain seems better adapted for navigating you, or an object you are controlling, through three dimensions. The right is used for defining depth, dimension, shape and movement. It is involved more than the left when mentally rehearsing the look of an object unfolded in three dimensions.

Many boys seem to be better on tasks that involve mentally rotating an object or imagining objects unfolded in three dimensions. They may be good at imagining their way around a large object like a ship, or a nuclear power station or a medieval castle. They certainly enjoy construction in three dimensions. I can personally testify to having cut out a dozen or so African animals from the back of cornflake packets by the age of ten. Sometimes before the cornflakes were eaten. They hung in the trophy room by the fireplace at the bottom of my bed. The publisher Dorling Kindersley had a fabulously popular series of books of cut-aways of ships, planes, spacecraft – even humans.

Boys are generally better at target-directed motor skills and interception: catching and throwing using gross motor movements. This is not an absolute. I can remember secretly admiring girls who were adept at hopscotch and who were also good at throwing and catching tennis balls against a wall in sequence with both hands, sometimes three at a go. The balls moved in a blur, the exercise was accompanied by a song and at the end of each verse another girl would jump in and take over the throwing and catching.

Girls do better on precision manual tasks such as peg boarding. Fine movement of the fingers is not fully co-ordinated in young children until about the age of five and it tends to be later in boys. In the great wars of the twentieth century, British women were recruited into munitions work and were particularly good at the speedy and accurate manipulation required for the assembly of bullets. I worked for a short period in a woollen mill. I worked in the dye house: all heavy lifting, heat, steam and men. In carding and spinning: all delicate fibres, noise, tying broken threads and women. The Purdue Pegboard looks like an old-fashioned cribbage board. It was designed to help in the recruitment of factory workers for intricate assembly-line work during the Second World War and involves the speedy manipulation of light metal pegs and washers into the holes on the board. Women always outperform men on the pegboard test.

Doreen Kimura, a Canadian-based researcher, and others[155] argue that women are better at controlling distal musculature – muscles further from the trunk. She and others also claim that in addition to being better at precise control such as replicating finger-tip touching patterns women are also better at co-ordinating several movements together.

This may come as no surprise to many women who are familiar with the notion of multi-tasking, but may disappoint men who think that, by right, they are better at driving a car, manipulating a tape into the tape player, holding a conversation on a mobile phone (illegally) that is trapped between neck and chin while looking for a road sign to get them off the M6.

Without any trace of irony, Kimura goes on to write, 'men, however, tend to be better at performing a single movement, such as tapping one key repeatedly with the same finger'. The next time you try to wean your son away from his Playstation 2 be aware you are fighting with destiny!

Some argue that the left hemisphere is more active with movements that are open loop and the right with closed loop. An open-loop movement is one that requires no correction or fine adjustment based on sensory feedback: sawing, turning the starting handle of an engine, stirring soup. Closed-loop movements are slower, modified regularly, adjusted by feedback: playing a snooker shot, typing, playing an instrument, throwing a ball. Kimura showed that an important function of the left side of the brain was to control the sequencing of articulatory movements of the mouth and tongue and of changes in limb posture. Damage to the left side of the brain can mean that patients recognize sequences of movement but cannot make them. When you smile you do so unevenly! For verbal and non-verbal movements, the right side of your mouth opens wider and faster. For emotions, the left side of your face is most expressive! It is controlled by the right hemisphere.

When right- and left-handers get into conversation they make different types of gestures. Left- and right-handers are equally likely to make self-touching gestures with both hands. Right-handers make more open gestures – movements with hands or arms away from the body – with their right hand than left-handers. Why? Doreen Kimura and others believe it is to do with centres for speech specialization and with sequencing articulatory movements being in the left hemisphere.

Chapter 12

Memory:

how do we remember?

This chapter contains the following sections:

⚶ **Thinking allowed**
Priming, context and cues in thought and recall. The difference between priming and cueing. Memory research using divers and using music.

⚶ **You forget for a purpose**
Forgetting is part of an effective memory. What happens when your memory is 'perfect'. False memory syndrome. Why each memory is an act of reconstitution.

⚶ **The mechanics of memory**
Memories are formed through a process of chemical and electrical change known as long-term potentiation. A break-through discovery in memory.

⚶ **Three parts of the brain used in memory**
A model of memory. The role of the amygdala, hippocampus and frontal cortex in memory formation and recall.

⚶ **Short and long: the systems of memory**
Different systems of memory. How information transfers from short-term memory to long-term. How much information can you store?

⚶ **Place, space 'n' face**
Research with London taxi drivers. Why you are good at remembering faces. How school children used visual memory to make dramatic improvements in SATs tests.

⚶ **Put on your memory SPECS**
A technique for improving recall that is over 2,000 years old. A simple memory tool for you or your students. Is there a place for rote learning?

... and will answer the following questions:

- ▷ Why does an answer to a question come to me when I am not expecting it?

- ▷ In self-help books I read, 'You have a perfect memory – if you know how to use it'. Is this true?

- ▷ What is a memory? Does it exist somewhere in the brain?

- ▷ Why do some people lose their memory? How does brain damage affect memory?

- ▷ I read a telephone number, I go to dial it and before I do so I have forgotten it. Why?

- ▷ Does your brain grow with use?

- ▷ What is the best way to remember anything?

Introduction

My great-great-grandmother was, according to my mother, a Scots Highland 'seer'. This meant that she had a sixth sense and would occasionally rule on some issue of family destiny. This also meant she got the best chair in the house and no one dared challenge her word. She would sit brooding in the corner by the fireplace with a furrowed brow and a slightly pungent aroma. From time to time she would utter some cryptic and necessarily gloomy judgement, 'yon bairn will ne'er hae a frosty pow'. This was said in reference to my mother's newly born cousin who later, as a merchant seaman in the last war, lost his life when his ship was bombed: he never reached old age, never had grey hair – did 'ne'er hae a frosty pow'.

Mind and memory must surely be more than the sum of the parts of electrical and chemical connections between neurons. Consciousness research, because of its controversial and beguiling nature, attracts disparate disciplines all offering radically different perspectives. So too does memory research. Memory research has benefited a great deal in recent years from multiple perspectives. What is and what is not memory? How do memories form and fail to form? What role does forgetting play in memory and is it essential for a good memory? Memory is not only what is consciously recalled and reconstituted, it is what is inhibited rather than erased. Memory 'loss' may also be an important part of creativity: remembering too much detail prevents you from seeing the pattern. Memory, like my great-great-grandmother's intuitive insights, may operate on the edges of conscious awareness, suddenly coming together as a result of an accumulation of previously unnoticed cues, available to some of us but only for some of the time. Our starting point in looking at the brain and memory is to look at the role of intuitive learning and at the value of forgetting.

Do you need to be conscious of an experience in order to learn from it? Can learning occur without conscious awareness? If there is such a thing as unconscious learning, how would we know that it had occurred? Would there be an ideal development stage for it? What circumstances would need to be in place for it to occur?

Thinking allowed

I borrowed my partner's car to go shopping. A rare event on a number of counts. I found myself afterwards in the car park of a very large shopping mall looking for my car. I could not find it. The shopping trolley wheels were almost ground to nothing by the time I gave up. I decided to sit down and take a breather, at which point a car drove by with two shopping bags on its roof. The shopping bags sitting there upright and on their own seemed absurd. I was unable to help. The car drove off. It was at that point, having been diverted from my preoccupation, that I realized I had been looking for my own car, but I had come in my partner's car. I found it straight away.

I believe that my narrowing preoccupation with limited data – my car and what it looks like – had inhibited me from thinking more broadly and remembering the important cues. A diversion had re-adjusted the focus for me.

Priming is also part of the process of recall. Priming can be loose or tight, direct or indirect. When it is direct – someone defines the category for us – or it can be indirect – the shopping bags on the car roof.

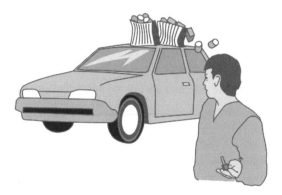

12.1 Narrowed thinking leaves the author carless. It takes a paradigm shift involving bags of shopping to solve the problem.

With recall, there is danger in priming too tight a set of categories to draw information from. Learning is about seeking and securing connections. Prime too narrowly and you do not get the connections. What does the word 'green' evoke in you? For me it is the face of a boy with whom I went to school. For you, it may be the meadow in the centre of the village near your house. What does it mean to a professional snooker player? It may mean the ball by the cushion next to the last red. What does it mean to a professional golfer? Hit it first time or we go home with no prize money!

Creativity and breadth of thought can be stifled by priming that is too narrow. Lots of categories for recall seem better than too few. However, you have to watch the categories: more categories require harder thinking. Or do they?

The theory of 'flow' suggests that for creativity, 'the best thing to do to engage creatively is to stop thinking about it'. By doing so, other items from other categories are more likely to be evoked. In the brain, the inhibitory effects of stimulating the links between brain cells declines more quickly than excitatory. Flow involves willingly suspending disbelief. Edison is attributed with the quote, 'If you want to have a good idea, have lots of good ideas'. For Professor Nick Rawlins of the University of Oxford, 'thinking evokes priming, in other words, other items in the category are more likely and subsequently to be evoked and the more focused the priming, the more narrow the relatedness of concepts simply because it is close'.[156] Professor Guy Claxton of the University of Bristol describes the mechanics of the process in terms of 'an excitatory neural epicentre surrounded by inhibitory corralling'.[157] Memory is the potential for connections to be made. Corral our access routes too tightly and we inhibit creativity. Open the categories too loosely and we ask for a higher level of effort.

We can learn implicitly and do so by being cued by phenomena at the periphery of our senses. As we have discussed earlier, complex rules can be learned via exposure to sequences that adhere to the rules, without having any explicit notion of the rules or having learned them.[158]

Surprisingly, some findings from brain research run counter to what intuitively 'feels' like good teaching practice. Retrieval of memory can occur at a phenomenally fast rate. Professor Steven Rose, of the Brain and Behaviour Research Group at the Open University, describes the activation sequence in the brain as a particular memory is retrieved. Activation of the visual cortex occurs within 100 milliseconds, then within 300 milliseconds the frontal cortex, by 600 milliseconds Broca's area, then, as a choice is made, by 900 milliseconds there is activation in the right parietal cortex. The speed with which this can occur suggests that decisions can, and do, get made outside of conscious attention. There is, for example, a great deal of learning that goes on outside of conscious attention. The brain processes information that is 'neither attended to nor noticed' and this process is pervasive and ongoing. Children can, in some situations, be learning without the involvement of the teacher!

What is the significance of this for learning? The teacher may well have to stop mid-sentence when the words 'you'll never learn unless you pay attention' begin to be said. For some types of learning we can speed the process by cueing.

Memories are often context dependent. Restore the context and you reconstitute the memory. Vivid contexts are good for learning because they are rich in cues, but changing the context can be enough to ensure recall. Alan Baddeley of the University of Bristol taught two groups of volunteers long lists of words.[159] The first group learned the words in a classroom while the others learned them at the bottom of a swimming pool wearing the full scuba gear. Recall was then tested for both groups. Baddeley found that those who learned in the classroom remembered better in the classroom while those who learned underwater remembered better underwater. Proving what? Context is useful in shaping recall. Restore or approximate the original context and recall improves.

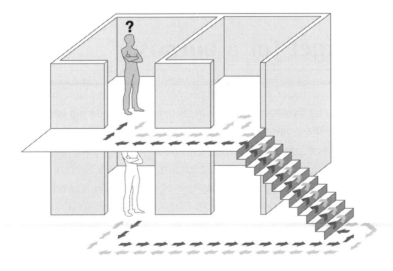

12.2 A context contains cues that can precipitate connections and allow recall to occur. Cues can be conscious or unconscious and accessed mentally or physically. Going from one room to another takes ten seconds. On arrival you discover you have forgotten what you came for. What do you instinctively do?

Using music can provide an important contextual cue in improving recall. Subjects in a context experiment viewed a list of words, one at a time. Two days later, they were given a test in which they simply had to recall as many of the learned words as possible. Like Baddeley's divers, learning and recall took place in the same or different context, but in this case the contexts were musical. There were three conditions during learning for different groups: a Mozart piano concerto (K491 in C), a jazz piece ('People Make the World Go Around' by Milt Jackson) or a quiet background. During the recall test, groups were subdivided so that they received either the same music (or quiet) that was present during learning or different music (or quiet).

Recall was best when the music was the same during learning and recall rather than when the pieces were changed. Quiet during both times did not aid memory. The worst recall when musical context was changed was found to be due to a memory process, rather than to possible distraction. Music, used as part of learning, can enter into memory and aid recall, even when it is not consciously attended to.

You forget for a purpose

The *Guardian* newspaper ran an advertisement on UK television in the 1980s that showed a black youth running aggressively towards an old white man in a public street. There was fear on the old man's face. The youth ran straight at him and pushed him violently to the ground. Both fell together, the youth on top of the old man. Then, almost simultaneously, a section of a wall crashed down onto where the old man had been standing seconds before. A voice-over said, 'Don't take things at face value.' At least that is how I remember it. But I may be wrong. As they say, 'Of all the liars, memory is the smoothest.'

Forgetting is part of an effective memory. At the molecular and cellular level in the brain, memory is highly dynamic. Memory is not fixed. If your memory was 'perfect', how miserable your life would be! Solomon Shereshevski, the world's most celebrated memory man, could memorize strings of numbers just by glancing at a blackboard. He performed memory feats for a living, recalling strings of numbers backwards or forwards months and years later.

Assessed for 30 years by the Russian psychologist Alexander Luria, Shereshevski complained that he could only remember things by picturing them and this hindered his mental capacity. His mind never developed beyond that of an adolescent because he could not think in the abstract. His mind was entombed in clutter. He could remember the numbers 2315 3166 4567 5678 but could not, no matter how hard he tried, see any sort of pattern.

Shereshevski could remember anything with amazing detail because he did so through the confused sensory system he was born with. His synaesthesia meant that he 'heard' colours, 'saw' tastes, 'felt' sounds, 'smelled' shapes! He would also detail the perceptions surrounding his memory feats, 'the colour feels rough and unpleasant, and it has an ugly taste … you could hurt your hand on this'. What sounds very confusing is actually a clue to an excellent way of encoding memory. By deliberately 'conflating' the physical qualities of the experience we make them more memorable. Shereshevski would also deploy a pegging technique to help him retrieve memories. He would imagine a series of facts in relation to a town that he had created for this purpose in his head. The town had features that were highly familiar to him: streets, houses, private homes, public buildings and facilities, meeting places and so on. When he was given a new fact he would associate it with a feature of the town and do so in a highly synaesthetic way: 'I smell the date which is on the flag of the Town Hall by the brightly coloured square' thus two memory techniques – pegging and synaesthesia – are combined.

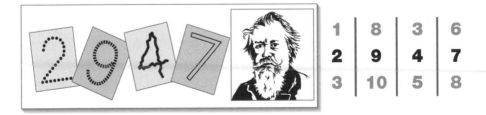

12.3 Solomon Shereshevski had a near-perfect memory for particular types of information. His memory was pictorial and synaesthetic. He was poor at context and discerning pattern. He was also deeply unhappy.

One in four of us are susceptible to false memory syndrome. With prompting and coaxing, one in four of us can be led to believe that something has occurred in our past that, in fact, has no basis in truth. Each year in the United States 77,000 people are charged with crimes based solely on eyewitness evidence and, according to the US National Institute of Justice figures for 1999, there are five who have been sentenced to death on eyewitness testimony alone. In Holland, after the 1992 Amsterdam plane crash, a study showed that an impossible 66 per cent of those interviewed claimed to have seen the event. Witness testimony is vulnerable to suggestibility and in particular there are differences of reliability with regard to age, race, presence of a weapon and duration of exposure to the evidence. Older people are more likely to pick someone from an identity parade. Own race bias (ORB) means that the identification of someone of one's own race is more accurate than someone of another race. In the presence of a weapon an eyewitness focuses in a tunnelled way on the weapon and not on the person at the other end of it.[160] Successful bank raids with carrots and aubergines prove this!

It can be seen that memory is a more malleable phenomenon than everyday sense would lead us to believe. This makes the 'truth' itself more fallible, particularly when it involves an individual drawing upon it. In order for us to survive and to lead balanced and healthy lives, we have become accomplished practitioners in false memory syndrome. Thankfully this is a very necessary part of everyday existence: a survival imperative. What would your life be like if you could remember everything?

In truth each memory is an act of reconstitution. The process of recall is influenced by many variables including emotional state, physiological condition, context and how this memory may connect with others. The same event can never be remembered exactly as it was. Every recall is a reconstitution and so plays its part in slightly distorting the original.

In some cases we cannot remember because the memory was not encoded as worthy enough of recall in the first place. We failed to give it serious significance so it never hit our radar. Some scientists believe that many memories are simply put out of everyday reach. This would be useful because it would not cause confusing clutter. This process is known as inhibition. People like Shereshevski are believed to have poor inhibitory mechanisms.

Not being able to forget can affect your health. Quite aside from the constant reliving of a traumatic experience, the bane that is PTSD (post traumatic stress disorder), being unable to inhibit can lead to depression. People who tend to mull things over excessively experience longer periods of depression than those who do not. Inhibiting uses up mental resources. People with lower IQ scores are more likely to suffer from PTSD and from extended depression. Perhaps this is to do with less working memory being available for dampening down unwanted recollections.

In memory work it is important to distinguish between measures of recognition and measures of recall. Multiple choice tests and true/false choices prompt recognition. Essay-type responses demand recall. It is also important for us to understand that memory is complex, messy, changing, multi-layered and imperfect. It is designed to be. Do not be seduced by those who promise that 'your memory is perfect – if only you know how to use it'. It is designed to be imperfect! If it were otherwise, life would be a never-ending nightmare of data tumbling out and at us.

The mechanics of memory

At the smallest level in the brain, memories are formed through a process of chemical and electrical change known as long-term potentiation or LTP. Long-term potentiation is the mechanism, neurologists believe, through which memories are encoded and so become capable of recovery.

At the cellular level in the brain, each and every new experience causes some neurons to connect and others to deteriorate. Little chemical and electrical messengers are sent on their way from one neuron to another. The more this happens the more they connect and the more others neglect. It is a form of natural selection. The more neural connections are reinforced, the more alternative connections are neglected. A single one of your neurons produces almost a tenth of a volt and the total electrical activity in your brain is easily measurable with an EEG.

The connections take the form of small electric charges. Patterns form and these patterns become raw material of memory. The patterns represent the

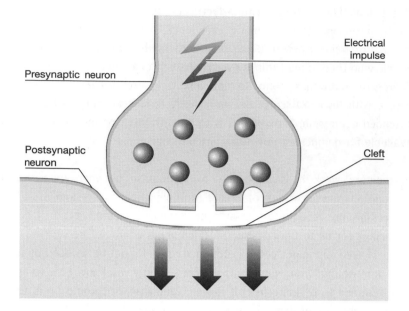

12.4 Mind the Gap. Long-term potentiation is a long-lasting increase in the efficacy of a synapse. Proteins produced in the first neuron must find their way to specific synapses and bind to them. This changes the structure of the synapses and permanently increases their sensitivity to an incoming signal.

initial memories associated with the experience. If and when the pattern of connections is re-activated, a process known as potentiation begins to occur. This makes subsequent connections easier and more likely. The process of becoming more permanent is known as long-term potentiation or LTP. From what we know of LTP we could argue a strong case that learning acts as exercise for the brain. 'A brain accustomed to being intellectually stretched will have more blood capillaries to help carry oxygen and glucose, more supportive glial cells, more all-round capacity to meet the metabolic and nutritional demands of the brain's neurons.'[161] What should happen with a period of extended lethargy? If neurons in the sequence are allowed to weaken, then the memory weakens. If we do not use it, then we live with the possibility of losing it. John Ratey describes it like this,

> An initial stimulation triggers a communication across the synapse between two nerve cells in the brain. Further stimulation then causes the cells to produce key proteins

that bind to the synapse, cementing the memory in place. If LTP – and hence a memory – is to last for more than a few hours, proteins produced in the first neuron must find their way to specific synapses and bind to them, an event that changes the structure of the synapses and increases their sensitivity to an incoming signal. This process may explain the need for rehearsal in learning as well as the value of REM sleep.[162]

LTP is the most compelling of explanations for the workings of memory. To use a horticultural analogy, it is akin to hacking clear a path and then walking that pathway. Neglect the pathway and it becomes overgrown. Use the pathway and it remains a viable communications route and is easier for every subsequent journey.

Antonio Damasio describes the process of memory along the lines of 'convergence zones'.[163] Convergence zones are the points that are physically near the sensory neurons that first registered the event. Professor Susan Greenfield talks of this in terms of 'promiscuous neurons gathered together in assemblies'.[164] This is a bit like ripples in a pond moving out and from time to time hitting other ripples from a different source

Damasio, who has used MRI as part of his research, also proposes a hierarchy of convergence zones. Lower convergence zones link the cues that allow us to understand the general concept of 'dog', while higher convergence zones allow us to recognize specific 'dogs'. Linking the two may be convergence zones that are used to recognize different elements of the dog – tail, head, coat – and then specific types of dog.

Does a sea slug have good memory? What about a fruit fly? Both are being used in breakthrough research into the mechanics of memory. Given that it may not have a very long life, a fruit fly has a surprisingly useful memory. Recent research with fruit flies suggests that short-term memory utilized proteins that are present at the synapses.[165] Long-term memory required a different process. To shift the memory into the long term, new proteins that re-configure synapses are needed. This synthesis is controlled by a protein known as CREB. CREB acts like a switch to trigger production of new proteins or turn it off. CREB has two opposing functions – one is to activate and the other is to suppress. The activator promotes long-term memory formation; the repressor impairs the memory.

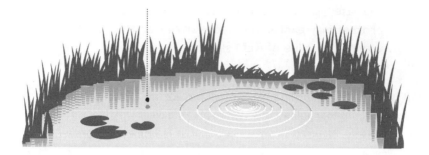

12.5 Neurons send out signals to others clustered nearby and they, in turn, respond and send on or return the signal. The effect is like ripples in a pond.

In the fruit fly study, scientists found that they could either speed up the formation of memories or block them by altering the levels of repressor and activator. Normally, following ten training sessions with a short rest in-between each one, fruit flies retain the information that an odour signals an electric shock is on its way. Flies with extra activator remembered more effectively. One lesson was enough for them. Flies that over-produced the repressor, however, could not form a specific long-term memory, even after many training sessions.

Researchers found that alterations of activator and repressor levels also affected mice memory when they had to complete complex tasks. In one test, mice had to rely on lasting memories to find a hidden dock in a pool of water. Those with lots of activator swam to the dock and stood on it easily. Those with repressor swam and swam without finding the dock. In another experiment, they had to choose a meal that matched the smell of a fellow mouse's breath. The mice with low levels of CREB activator could not remember the smell and so did not eat as well. The researchers pinpointed the hippocampus as one of the brain areas where CREB exerts its power. Mature rats had their CREB activity disrupted, solely in the hippocampus. They also showed a deficiency in long-term memory function.

Working with mice, Cold Spring Harbor Institute researcher Dr Alcino Silva discovered the importance of 'wait time' in learning. Mice improved their learning performance with short periods of rest during training sessions. The speculation is that the brain uses this time to recycle CREB.[166]

One of the outcomes of the CREB research is that scientists are testing a large number of existing drugs that may be able to enhance memory by affecting CREB in rodents.

Three parts of the brain used in memory

The brain has multiple memory systems for storing information. This has been known for many years. Patient H who suffered from epileptic seizures and had to have drastic surgery to separate the two halves of his brain has been locked into the moment ever since. His recall of the period of his life prior to his operation is intact. He believes he is still in the 1950s of his youth. If, however, you should visit him, he would not be able to remember your name or who you are by the end of a 20-minute conversation. Oliver Sacks, a clinical neurologist, describes in detail how patients whom he treated suffered unusual aberrations in memory as a result of illness.[167]

One man who came to him was a music teacher, who during the first office visit faced Sacks with his ears, not his eyes. His gaze seemed 'unnatural, darting and fixating' on the doctor's features one at a time. He had come with his wife who sat throughout the interview. When it finished the man appeared to grasp his wife's head and try to lift it off and put it on his own head. 'He had, as Sacks says, mistaken his wife for a hat!' The wife, in turn, gave no hint that something out of the ordinary had occurred!

A second interview took place at the man's home. He was unable to recognize the rose in Sacks's lapel, describing it as 'a convoluted red form with a linear green attachment'. Encouraged to speculate on what it might be, he guesses it could be a flower. When he smells it, he comes to life and knows it. His wife explains that her husband makes sense of everyday things through his senses.

He functions by making little songs about what he is doing – dressing, washing or eating and if the song is interrupted he has to stop. Then he waits until he finds a sensory clue on how to proceed. There is a site within the brain that contributes to facial recognition. Damage to it means that aberrant behaviours occur and the patient has to resort to other methods to perform simple recognition.

Memories of everyday episodes (episodic memory) use different brain structures from memories of facts and information (semantic memory). Some patients with profound amnesia cannot remember who you are a minute after you have introduced yourself but can talk on to you with relative ease. We use different areas for encoding memory and retrieving memory. It does not come out in the way it went in!

John Ratey is Associate Clinical Professor of Psychology at Harvard Medical School. He describes memory as, 'the centripetal force which pulls together, learning, understanding and consciousness'.[168] In talking about the brain and memory he goes on to say 'the brain is more like an active ecosystem than a static, pre-programmed computer. There is no single centre for vision, language, emotion, social behaviour, consciousness or ... memory'. This is a point worth reinforcing. There are no single centres in the brain in which specific memories are located. An act of re-membering is like a unique coming together. A family gathering for a wedding anniversary would be a better metaphor for understanding memory than a computer or a library or an archive. This is because memory is not static. The act of re-membering is part of the memory itself.

We cannot separate the act of retrieving from the memory itself. The memory in its quiescent state does not exist. It is as though, in our imaginary wedding anniversary, an invite is sent out to family members and friends and maybe a few other distant acquaintances. The family expect it and are primed for a quick response; the friends, surprised by the invitation, have to be prompted; you have to work much harder to contact that acquaintance of your father's whom he has not seen for thirty years. The memory is as much in the uniqueness of their coming as it is in the event itself. This is what it is like in your brain when it remembers.

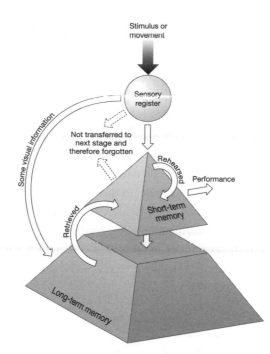

12.6 A model of memory. A physical experience registers as data where it is held for a short period. Its fading is like the decline of an echo. The information needs to be transferred out from the sensory register in order to be held. Some visual information goes to long-term memory directly. Some goes to short-term memory if we have attended to it and decided – at some level – it is needed. Once it is in short-term memory it needs rehearsal or application to transfer to long-term memory. Recall involves transferring back held data from long-term memory to short-term memory. Every act of retrieval is, in fact, a reconstitution so we never get back a verbatim transcript from long-term memory.

Three parts of the brain take a controlling function in memory. Their roles are like those needed to organize your parents' wedding anniversary celebrations. They are the amygdala, the hippocampus and the frontal cortex.

The amygdala decides the emotional value of the proposal. This is like deciding on how extravagant a celebration to hold. The amygdala is asking does this mean something to me? How significant is this to me? It then gives it an emotional 'tag' based on a significance reading. The 'tag' is like a value it is allocated. If the amygdala is maladapted as a result of some sort of trauma or dysfunction, it will affect the emotional valuation given to the experience. If your general emotional state is depressed or is artificially high, that alters the emotional value that is tagged to the memory. Brother and sister share the same parents but their 'experience' of being parented differs. They may tag the event of a wedding anniversary differently.

The amygdala is better at tagging negative emotional events, particularly those arousing fear or sadness, and they are better remembered than events with neutral emotional content. Observed while watching horror films, adults showed a surprising link between activity in the amygdala and the number of frightening events. What is fascinating about this is that it showed arousal of emotion in the brain, even when the subjects claimed not to be affected by the films in any way. It seems another area of the brain – the hippocampus – is more involved in remembering events that are emotionally more neutral.

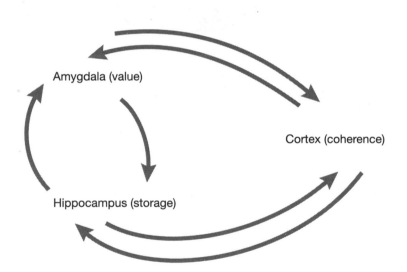

12.7 In retrieving memory the amygdala, hippocampus and frontal cortex are all involved. The amygdala assigns an experience an emotional 'value'. The hippocampus decides on where and how the information is stored. The cerebral cortex helps package the memory into a coherent whole.

Next, information is routed simultaneously to the hippocampus and the cortex. The hippocampus is in both hemispheres and it has a central role in re-membering. Memory may indeed be about dis-membering and then re-membering with the hippocampus central to both stages. In our extended metaphor of memory and wedding reception, the hippocampus seems to act like the person or family members who decide who should and who should not come. Not everyone is invited, not everyone is told. The hippocampus is deciding what information goes where. A proposal comes in, it is considered, evaluated, acted upon and the relevant contacts made. This is what the hippocampus is doing with the tagged information received from the amygdala.

The third area of simultaneous involvement is the frontal cortex. It acts like an overall planning executive that oversees the decisions being made about whom to invite to the celebrations. The frontal cortex is involved in planning, evaluating consequences and determining goals. The frontal cortex develops late and when damaged can lead to impulsive and reckless behaviour. In the brain, it is the frontal cortex that neatly organizes the pieces of memory into a temporal, logical and meaningful story.

You go from one room in the house to another to get something. You travel 3 metres, it takes four seconds and you have forgotten what you went in for. An explanation of this short-term memory phenomena will follow somewhere towards the end of this sentence, but in order to be able to understand it you need to remember the beginning until you arrive here, at the end. Make sense? It is what is sometimes referred to as 'working memory' that allows us to exist on a moment-by-moment basis. Working memory is part of the executive function of the pre-frontal cortex in the brain. Its essential feature is minute-by-minute decision making. Decisions are made on the basis of past experience. Working memory lends coherence to experience. Without it we would be enslaved to the trivia of each moment.

Working memory acts as a 'doorman' at the front gate of consciousness, allowing only certain valued experiences to be encoded. If this were not so, we would become habitual archivists, paralysed into any activity because of the constant bombardment of disconnected sensory data.

Work done by Elizabeth Loftus at the University of Washington in Seattle on planting false memories suggests about one in four of us believe them to be real.[169] As the original memory is 'recalled', the experience begins to feel real.

Later it will be this feeling of reality that will authenticate the memory. We recall the vague feeling of authenticity alongside the memory. We are then seduced into its 'truth'. According to Dr Daniel Wright, a psychologist working with the UK Eyewitness Research Unit, 'In 20 per cent of identity parades victims pick a person whom police know to be innocent.'[170] He is among many who believe that false memory, and thus wrongful conviction, is more prevalent than we think.

Wright conducted an experiment with 40 students looking at a picturebook that tells the story of a crime committed at a snooker hall. The book contains photographs of two men and a woman. The woman steals a wallet from one of the men. The students all look at the picturebook on their own, except half of the books have the woman loitering with an accomplice and the other have her on her own. No one knew there was any difference. When questioned afterwards on their own as to whether the woman had an accomplice 39 out of 40 gave an accurate response. Then the groups were put

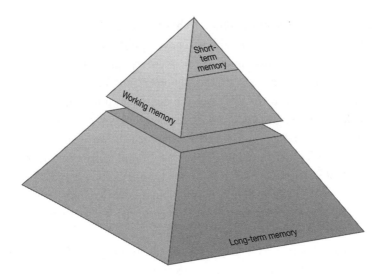

12.8 Working memory is a general term for all that is not long-term memory. Working memory allows us to exist on a moment-by-moment basis. It is part of the executive function of the pre-frontal cortex in the brain. It involves selection, deletion and distortion. It includes the sensory register. Short-term memory is a sub-set of working memory and is a temporary storage space for new information. Short-term memory can be limited by duration or by digit span.

into mixed pairs with each pair having someone who had seen the picturebook with the accomplice and someone who had seen the picturebook with no accomplice. They were then asked, what happened? None of the pairs ought to have reached agreement. Only four failed to reach an agreement. The rest compromised. Sixteen pairs persuaded themselves one way or another, with nine reporting no accomplice and seven reporting an accomplice. When we are given information we use it to fill gaps. Having someone describe an event is a powerful way of altering a memory.

So working memory involves a certain amount of selection, deletion and distortion. False memory is part of this. False memory syndrome is a distortion of a natural process. Memories can be planted. Give people a selection of childhood memories, three of which are real and one of which is false, and many respondents will come to believe with absolute certainty that all are real. Memory involves selection. Selection occurs at a number of levels, including conscious and unconscious levels. Memory involves dis-membering experience first and re-membering experience later. We store by similarity; we retrieve by difference.

Short and long: the systems of memory

Short-term memory is a sub-set of working memory and is like RAM – it is there while we need it but as soon as the computer is switched off we lose it. Short-term memory is largely defined by its susceptibility. When subjects were asked to hold new information while counting backwards from 100, recall of the new information consistently declined to zero after about ten seconds.

If you were asked to take a random sequence of numbers and repeat them back to me, how many would you be able to remember before you made an error? Try it from the list overleaf. Read out the numbers in sequence then close your eyes and pause before repeating the sequence. At what point do you make an error?

7324

4718

32901

51899

064528

348371

8137649

5633407

21440753

93057312

219843781

520791642

4852066738

65782179342

91524837623

This is a very crude measure of digit span. Interestingly it is influenced by the sounds that the number comprises. The longer the sounds, the more information the brain is asked to carry, the less efficient we may be at doing so. In languages where the sounds of numbers are shorter and more varied performance goes up. Most people in the West can manage about seven digits, some nine or ten and some only five or six. Try mixing numbers with letters or with letters and symbols. Recall is also influenced by method of rehearsal. Saying them aloud helps. Saying them in a rhythmic way also helps. Looking for patterns, chunking them down and visualizing them works to provide slight performance improvements.

Short-term memory needs some sort of meaningful activation for the temporary storage to become more permanent. Long-term memory is like putting it onto the hard drive so we can use it again and again. How does the conversion from short-term memory to long-term memory occur? What is the sequence of events in the brain?

Conversion does not occur until information is sent by the cortex to the hippocampus and research suggests there is a time space needed for this to happen. The space is the length of time it takes for the neurons to synthesize the necessary proteins for LTP. For learning, 'wait' or processing time is vital. For this reason educators ought to be good at facilitating 'waiting' after asking a question. The learner needs to hear the question, assimilate it, formulate a response and then surface the response in some way. Asking for too quick a response gets in the way of processing time.

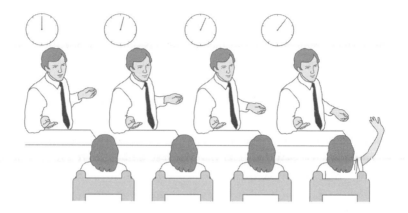

12.9 We need processing time when asked a question to hear the question, assimilate it and compare it to others that we have been asked, formulate a response from a possible range and surface the response in language. All of which takes time – processing time.

Good teachers give tools to encourage a wider range of categories in a learner's thinking. This is a form of processing time. They ask questions like: what alternatives should we also consider? How might someone else approach this problem? Let us think about this one upside down or back to front or inside out! One teacher I know approaches difficult problems by pretending she takes off her own head and physically puts on someone else's: how would the headteacher approach this? What about the chair of governors? What about a parent?

Sleep is also a form of processing time. But it has to be the right sort of sleep. Research done in Israel with laboratory rats discovered that the type of sleep also mattered in recall. Interrupting REM sleep again and again led to complete blockage of recall. Interruption of non REM sleep again and again did not.

Long-term memory is classified in a number of ways. The main distinction is declarative or procedural. Declarative memory includes episodic and semantic memory. Procedural includes motor memory and conditioned responses. Declarative memory is the 'what'. Procedural is the 'how'. Schools and formal education focus to excess on the 'what'. As humans we are naturally better at doing the 'how'.

Declarative memory includes both episodic and semantic types of recall. Episodic memory is memory of the 'moment' and is time tagged. With episodic memory, you remember the experience and its circumstances. Memory and the structures that are activated in recall is distributed throughout the brain but types of memory have high dependency on certain areas.

Semantic memory is the memory of meanings and of related information, facts and figures, faces, places and things. These data are directly accessible to our conscious awareness. Semantic memory is not necessarily connected to a time or a place. The fact that you remember that Paris is the capital of France is not necessarily linked to the first time you discovered this. Semantic memory is rapidly retrievable when effectively rehearsed, unreliable when poorly rehearsed. It involves both the cortex and the hippocampus. Some Alzheimer's patients lose declarative memory including names, places, faces, facts, their own identity but retain procedural skills such as knitting. Amnesiacs often acquire motor skills at a rapid rate and often quicker than those with an unimpaired memory. They retain such procedural memories when the memory of everyday facts is lost.

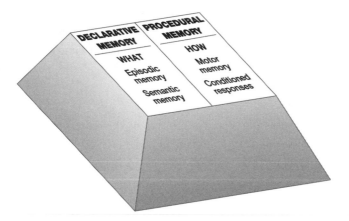

12.10 The main distinction is between declarative or procedural, declarative being the 'what', procedural the 'how'. Declarative memory includes episodic and semantic memory, procedural includes motor memory and conditioned responses.

Procedural memory includes your recall of a sequence of steps. For example, the recall of habits and skills that, once rehearsed thoroughly, do not have to be consciously accessed: walking, throwing, catching, riding a bicycle. They are slowly retrieved, inflexible and thoroughly reliable. They involve the basal ganglia and cerebellum, both involved in the control of movement. Eventually you do not go through each step in conscious awareness nor do you need to, as it has been sufficiently rehearsed to go from explicit to implicit. Learning includes the ready ability to turn declarative learning – specifically explicit memory – into procedural learning and, specifically, implicit memory. As a skill is moved from explicit to implicit, then its location in the brain changes. Research into brain disorders such as Parkinson's disease, which affects the basal ganglia, shows that declarative memory can remain intact while some procedural memory goes. Sufferers can understand who they are, remember their past, know facts and figures and recognize faces but struggle to make a series of habituated movements such as walking or talking.

The development of semantic memory is similar in some ways to the development of motor memory. Both benefit from distributed rehearsal. New information and skills become stored in long-term procedural memory with rehearsal. The best sort of rehearsal is distributed. In other words, practise a little and often. According to Dr Larry Cahill, of the University of California at Irvine, this prevails throughout the 'learner kingdom', 'from fruit flies to humans, distributed learning works better than amassed learning and so adding more content comes at a price'.[171]

Place, space 'n' face

Visual long term memory has been described as a 'special case in humans'. We are really good at remembering places, spaces and faces.

Studies with children show that they have photographic-like recall for visual memory until about the age of six by which time most have been to school for about a year. Anthropologists studying peoples without written language talk of their photographic-like ability to recall objects and places. How old is the act of reading? Written language evolved among humans some 10,000 years ago, 90,000 years after the human brain had evolved to its present form. The phenomenal capacity we have for visual recall reflects our evolutionary history. We are naturally good at remembering the look of things and their spatial relationships.

Dominic O'Brien is the current and eight-times winner of the World Memory Championships. He can recall 40 decks of cards and has done so against the clock with only one mistake, 100 names and faces learned in half an hour, a 500-word poem in 15 minutes and a deck of cards in 36 seconds. He is not a freak! He decided only 14 years ago to train his memory and now makes a living from it. How does he do it? One of the methods he uses involves physical locations. He has in his head, should he need them, 80 pre-learned possible journeys with 52 stops each.[172] He has little difficulty navigating the pre-rehearsed sequence of stops and at each he quickly makes exaggerated associations with the new information. He assigns the unfamiliar to the familiar and organizes it via a visual and spatial sequence.

You use visual memory to navigate, to recall the physical location and shape of objects and to manoeuvre yourself or objects in space. Visuo-spatial memory is imperative for survival and always has been. At its most sophisticated, it is James Bond recognizing his enemy's position by tracking the slow movement of his shadow. It is the same sophistication that a homing pigeon uses to find its one metre coop from 650 kilometres away. It is the same sophistication that allows you to recognize that the lines of colour on a Picasso canvas in front of your face represent the consequences for a nation of a bombing raid that occurred over 60 years ago.

Patients with Alzheimer's can suffer from two forms of visuo-spatial memory impairment. They depend on the location of lesions. Lesions in the right hemisphere inhibit patients' ability to understand the Big Picture. At the circus, they would see the clown's large shoes, the star on the elephant's head, the chalk on the trapeze artist's hands but not be able to make sense of it all. Lesions in the left hemisphere inhibit patients' ability to understand the particulars. They would see the brightly coloured tent, the audience, experience the excitement and laughter but not appreciate what was happening and why.

A growing field of research suggests that there are specific genes that are responsible for place memory. Some of us may be better disposed to spatial recall than others. Dr Tsusumu Tonegawa at MIT discovered a gene responsible for long-term episodic memory. His work, along with that of Eric Kandel at Columbia University, showed that this gene, in the hippocampus, is responsible for 'place' memory only, not other types too. When this gene is enhanced, rats show an amazing photographic memory, resulting in one time learning. Without it, they are lost and take 20 or more trials for the same result.[173]

In a London school, children were encouraged to look at key information through learning posters placed around the classroom. This was part of an accelerated learning initiative at the school. The posters contained limited amounts of chunked information and were easy to read and to see. Children were encouraged to test their recall of the 'look' of each content poster, to draw them in exercise books, to 'teach' them to others and to try to draw them from memory. At the end of the year the children's performance improvement in their standardized tests was among the highest in the country. They could remember the look of key information and its spatial relationship with what surrounded it. In a wonderful moment of serendipity, neuroscience explained why the following year.

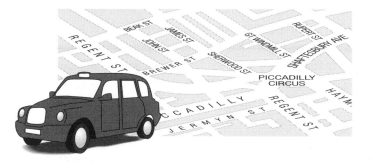

12.11 Evidence that there can be structural changes in healthy human brains was provided by research into London taxi drivers. Part of the hippocampus grew larger as the taxi drivers spent more time in the job.

In September 2000 I was travelling in a taxi to Paddington station from the Institute of Cognitive Neuroscience in London. I had been to a seminar on neuroscience and learning and I had sneaked out early. It does not always happen like this in London but I got talking to the driver on amicable terms.

He asked me what I had been doing there. I told him. He told me a story of how he could remember customers by associating them with places. For example, he had dropped off a student at the Institute two years before. This was only one of two occasions he had been there. She was a tea drinker and a sociology student. He told me he remembered this because he had picked her up again, about a year later, and asked her if she was still drinking tea. As she had only just got into the cab and not said anything, she was taken aback and later said as much. How could he have remembered all that time later? This was interesting, and I told him about the University College research released earlier that year on London taxi drivers' brains.

In tests conducted with 15 London taxi drivers, some of whom had over 40 years' experience, it was found that their brains had adapted to help them hold a map of the city in their heads. The research team lead by Dr Eleanor Maguire[174] used MRI techniques and compared the brains of taxi drivers with 50 others in a control group. They found that the taxi drivers had a larger hippocampus compared to control groups and that part of the hippocampus grew larger as they spent more time in the job.

The tests found the only area of the taxi drivers' brains that was different from the 50 other 'control' subjects was the left and right hippocampus. 'The hippocampus has changed its structure to accommodate their huge amount of navigating experience. One particular region of the hippocampus, the posterior or back, was bigger in the taxi drivers,' said Dr Maguire. The front of the hippocampus was smaller in the taxi drivers compared to the controls. 'This is very interesting because we now see there can be structural changes in healthy human brains.'

The posterior hippocampus was also more developed in taxi drivers who had been in the career for 40 years than in those who had been driving for a shorter period.

'There seems to be a definite relationship between the navigating they do as a taxi driver and the brain changes,' said Dr Maguire. One exciting consequence of this research is that it provides evidence that the brain is able to change physically according to the way it is used. This could have important implications for people with brain damage or brain diseases such as Parkinson's. For a long time it has been felt that there was only a limited amount of plasticity in the adult brain. Perhaps rehabilitation programmes in the future could utilize this kind of knowledge?

The taxi driver who picked me up from the Institute and I started to talk about the 'knowledge'. He told me it takes, on average, about four years to 'learn' London and the suburbs. He had done it in 17 months. This was very unusual, so I asked him what he had done to learn the information so quickly. He was a Cockney, he had a moped and he had been ill. All of which was relevant to his success. He used lots of rhyming slang in everyday speech and was good at manipulating language sounds. He remembered by rehearsing the sounds of street names in his head. He used acronyms – Chelsea, Albert and Battersea bridges became CAB. Then he became ill. This meant he was confined to bed, at first in hospital and then at home, for several weeks. During this time he pored over the maps and the A–Z of London and mentally rehearsed the routes in his head, again and again. If you visit London, you will see lots of very large men on very small mopeds in the most obscure streets. Attached to their handlebars is a plastic map holder. They are physically rehearsing the knowledge by getting out and doing it.

How long would it take you to do the knowledge? The knowledge is perfect recall of all of central London and the suburbs, streets and landmarks as well as places of interest, galleries, museums, theatres, hotels and restaurants. London taxi drivers have to demonstrate that they have the knowledge before they are licensed to drive a cab in London. If you had taken a leaf out of my taxi driver's book and learned by hearing, seeing and doing, then, I would suggest, you would do it a lot quicker than by simple rote.

When we remember faces, we do so with different parts of the brain. Working memory can transfer information to long-term memory within 60 seconds of encoding and, as we age, we rely more and more on the left pre-frontal cortex and less on the right visual cortex. As soon as something is experienced we interpret and thus re-wire the memory. Rather than remember the visual image, we use the associations, thoughts and impressions associated with the face. The implication of this finding is that even as we attempt to describe information held in working memory we are using different structures of the brain to do so. Thus every memory is an act of reconstitution. We make it up as we go along!

When you see an attractive face, sites that are also associated with reward become active. Knut and Kampe, of the Institute of Cognitive Neuroscience at University College, London, asked 16 volunteers to rate 40 different unknown faces as attractive.[175] They were asked to look for qualities such as radiance, empathy, cheerfulness and even motherliness, as well as conventional beauty. While their brains were scanned they were asked to rate the attractiveness of each face on a scale of one to ten. Faces deemed attractive by the subject, irrespective of gender, activated a certain part of the brain. This only happened when there was eye contact, not when the pictures showed an averted gaze. The part of the brain activated is the ventral striatum, the brain's reward centre. Studies in monkeys and rats have shown that this part of the brain lights up on anticipation of a reward such as food or water. It is also involved in addiction. The research also shows that an attractive face is recognized by the brain in a matter of seconds. This suggests it is an automatic process, perhaps hard-wired into the brain.

Our ability to recognize faces is remarkable. Our faces are very similar. Yet we can instantly tell whether a face we see before us is a friend, a relative or a complete stranger. The apparently simple task of recognizing a face actually takes up a huge amount of processing power. The task is so brain-intensive, in fact, that our facial recognition system only works with faces that are the right way up. Notice how much more quickly you recognize the faces that are the right way up than the faces that are upside down.

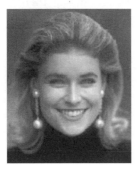 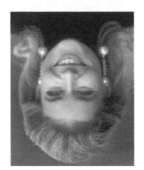 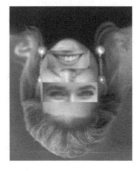

12.12 Three faces. One the right way up, another upside down and another upside down apart from the eyes and mouth.

Ralph Haber collected thousands of slides of faces and places and at the rate of one per second spent a morning session showing them to his psychology students.[176] The slides contained images of people and of locations in and around the area where Haber lived. The students would not have recognized them. A couple of days later he showed the same slides, but each now shown alongside a new slide randomly positioned left or right. Asked to say which was the original slide from a population of now over two thousand, there was a 90 per cent accuracy rate. Without any practice or rehearsal the visual information had somehow been secured in long-term memory. We are really good at doing this sort of thing and yet many learning environments and many textbooks are bereft of visual cues.

Put on your memory SPECS

Techniques for improving memory are surprisingly enduring. The methods used nowadays in expensive management seminars are no different from methods used in Greek or Roman times. The basic message is I, F and R. This means Intent, File and Rehearse. Decide on what is important to recall (by doing so you give it significance), then store it through some mechanism (for example, using mnemonics or association) and then rehearse (go over it until you are comfortable in being able to access it in a variety of situations). The methods taught on management courses focus on stage two – File – and are variations on ways of giving information significance.

To make something memorable put on your memory specs! Focus on what it is you wish to remember then: see it, personalize it, exaggerate it, connect it and then share it – SPECS! Throughout, remember that experiences that have an emotional resonance get remembered best – so really go for it!

What follows is a basic memory improvement package in a paragraph. It is a descriptor of a process. Pay attention at the back! Motivation is important in recall. Here goes.

Tag the experience as significant by deciding what it is you want to remember. **Prime** this by identifying what sort of information it is and how it connects to what you already know. **Sell** yourself the benefits of knowing this information. As a result of doing this how will I be better off? You have now given the activity of remembering significant attention and are ready to **encode**. To encode – or file – use the SPECS method: See the information, Personalize it, Exaggerate it, Connect it and Share it. Be consistent – if you rehearse in a particular place or in a particular way, it is easier if you continue to do it that way. To conclude, **rehearse** or go over the information frequently and **test**.

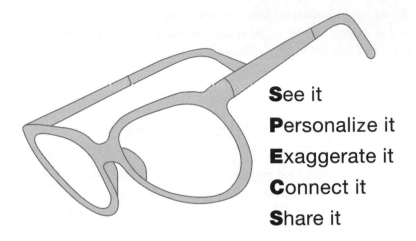

See it

Personalize it

Exaggerate it

Connect it

Share it

12.13 The SPECS memory filing technique. To enhance the likelihood of recall use the SPECS method: See the information, Personalize it, Exaggerate it, Connect it and Share it.

Finally, is there a place for rote learning? There is certainly value in distributed rehearsal and in spaced testing. Distributed rehearsal or a 'little and often' is fundamental to the maintenance of any skill. Recall scores go up with spaced testing. Rote learning is a sub-set of distributed rehearsal but with an emphasis on verbal familiarity. Separate fMRI studies looked at the brain response to rote repetition of vocabulary items. It was found that the areas of the brain used for speech production were also used for rote repetition. The significance of this is that with rote-learned material recall is prompted by verbal cues coded within speech networks.[177] Some believe that learners with poor neuronal capability for 'learning off by heart' can, nevertheless, learn through other means and brain imaging will, in time, reveal if this is the case. It is certain that capacity for learning things by rote is highly individualized.

For many young learners there is security in being able to demonstrate immediate knowing. Your child will feel esteemed by being able to recite their seven times table at the drop of a hat, but is it good use of neural real estate and limited class time? Rote learning does not invite us to understand connections. It does not open up alternative categories of knowledge. It does not deepen sensitivity to a poem's message. Nor does it give us insight to the application of maths. It does provide many learners with a set of tools that may have use over and above their immediate application.

As a child attending Sunday School in Scotland, I had to learn the books of the Old and New Testament in order from the King James Bible. What use has this been to me? Very little in everyday life, but maybe it has had some deeper value in reminding me that I can do it. Perhaps it has played a part in developing verbal fluency and a better understanding of patterns of sound and, most significantly, it has helped activate the neural circuitry for similar needs should they arise. Rote learning will always be controversial. It has its place. If I am on an international flight, I want the pilot to know the safety drill in the event of engine failure by heart. How it has been remembered is a different issue.

3
PART THREE
The brain's finally behind it

Chapter **13**

The findings

1 The outcomes of research into the workings of the human brain, particularly in the field of learning dysfunction, offer a great deal to educators. A lot of teaching that has been based on intuition and common sense could benefit from many of the informed insights neuroscience offers.

2 More effort is needed to convey research findings to educators accurately and intelligibly. At the moment there is no consistent mechanism through which this occurs. Without authoritative and informed insights the education community remains susceptible to glib truths – for example, the 10 per cent myth.

3 Monitoring for health is crucial in pregnancy and in the early years. More effective conduits to get information early to parents, especially about lifestyle choices and links to learning, are desirable.

4 The idea of the sensitive window is useful for the education community to know and understand. More work on the extent and duration of such windows – for example, do they exist for different areas of human endeavour – is needed. The concept of brain development being both dependent and expectant is also useful in reminding us of a balance between nature and nurture in learning.

▶▶❺ The brain has natural and separate circuits for language and for number. Development of such circuits start early. Children acquire and store language earlier than common sense dictates, provided there is repeated exposure to it. Exploration of the world of number starts in infancy and needs subsequent structured intervention.

▶▶❻ There is a need to invest in early years teaching but with a more informed and perhaps appropriate pedagogy. Hothousing, for far too many children, can be antagonistic to positive lifelong learning dispositions.

▶▶❼ A second – or any further – language needs to be taught early. Language acquisition favourably alters the structure of the brain. Is it worth the struggle to institutionalize language learning at a chronological phase when it has already become more difficult for the learner?

▶▶❽ It is vital to retain the motion and emotion components of learning: movement and music.

▶▶❾ Core skills and some factual information need to be taught. Teaching should utilize and align with what is known about brain development and structure. For example, teaching should provide structured challenge, multi-level engagement, imitation, aggregation and dis-aggregation, connections, real contexts and regular and reflective rehearsal.

▶▶❿ Respecting difference is less about badges of distinction – race, gender, disability – and more about accommodating different entry and exit points.

Chapter **14**

Recommendations

... for parents

1 Choose a lifestyle for learning. With the brain it is a case of use it or lose it. The brain circuitry developed in childhood provides the basis for all subsequent learning.

2 Monitor your lifestyle habits in pregnancy and when trying for a child. Poor diet, excess of stress, alcohol, nicotine, drugs all affect your child's brain.

3 The best care is 'kangaroo care'. In the early months particularly, 'skin to skin' helps contribute to emotional bonds between parent and child. This is a time when the child's stress response is being set for life.

4 Monitor your child's health and particularly hearing, eyesight and physical movement.

5 Play with your child and exploit mimicry and imitation. They are the first learning styles.

6 Harsh words alter a child's brain for life. Be constantly positive in the things you do and say with your child.

7 Be there to share. One of the greatest needs of a child is to share reactions with a consistent adult to a variety of outside stimuli.

Speak to, with and around your child from the earliest. Never underestimate an infant's capacity to store words.

 Be aware that the brain develops in spurts and plateaux and also that there are ideal times for certain learning experiences to occur.

 Avoid too formal too early. There is no real evidence that starting formal learning early advantages your child.

Recommendations

... for educators

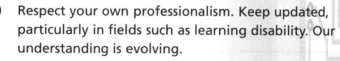

 Respect your own professionalism. Keep updated, particularly in fields such as learning disability. Our understanding is evolving.

 Multiple level engagement and global and local emphasis. Assume multiple entry and exit points in the design of your classroom learning activities. Always sit chunked information in a wider global context.

Scaffold challenge. Be aware that there is an emotional curriculum that lies below the surface and that those emotions direct attention. When a learner tips out of anxiety and into stress the behavioural response is predictable.

4 An understanding of both physical and physiological variables assists your teaching. Use variables such as the room, time on task and movement to help your learning outcomes. Be aware of the physiological state of the learners in front of you.

5 Model by proximity. Demonstrate through what you do and say. Be aware that learners need to approximate to a role model before they can adopt its practices. Too remote and it does not work.

6 Seek connections. At all levels and at all times, meaningful learning involves seeking and securing connections. An educator builds this into everyday classroom interactions

7 Optimize structured language exchange within each learning activity.

8 Teach and model the skills of memory.

9 Utilize processing time and build in reflective rehearsal.

10 Challenge naïve assumptions and easy truths about what the human brain is and is not. To do this you need to stay informed.

Recommendations
... for policy makers

1   Argue the case for more professional understanding of developmental stages of the human brain as part of Initial Teacher Training. Train more colleagues in dealing with learning disorders and in the early use of diagnostic tests.

2   Create a research community of educators and neuroscientists to share findings and 'cross the bridge' between scientific understanding and educational practice. Encourage educators to ask more specific questions of the science community with regard to learning.

3   Use the school as a learning lifestyle hub to revisit the concept of community education. Brain science tells us learning genuinely starts from 'in'spiration and only ends with 'ex'piration.

4   Informed parenting is key. Establish a 'parenting liaison' role with status to work within a core of trial schools and across community agencies.

5   Avoid push down of formal learning and replace with push down of dispositions learning: do so through more informed physical exploration and structured play in the early years.

6   Hold on to the arts provision, particularly music and movement.

7 Languages. Be bold enough to consider abandoning statutory languages teaching post-11 in favour of more interventions at an earlier age. Brain science supports this.

 8 Remove selection by test at 11. The developmental pattern of the immature brain means that such tests are unfair.

 9 Create a connections curriculum where all classroom and online learning has a philosophy of learning behind it and shows explicit connections to real contexts throughout.

10 Have the best brains in the country work on a funicular education system with multiple entry and exit points.

Chapter **15**

Questions

and where to find the answers

Chapter 16

Recommended websites

The author

www.alite.co.uk
Contact Alistair via his website!

Child development and prenatal care

www.allianceforchildhood.net/
Alliance for Childhood

www.nauticom.net/www/cokids/teacher
Early years and brain-based learning

www.cdi.page.com
The Child Development Institute

www.ich.ucl.ac.uk/
Institute of Child Health

www.hea.org.uk
Health Education Authority

www.nct-online.org
National Childbirth Trust

www.sheilakitzinger.com
Sheila Kitzinger, midwifery specialists' homepage

www.doh.gov.uk
UK Department of Health

Training and development organizations

www.brainconnection.com
Brain connection site

www.brain.com
Brain.com site

www.6seconds.org/
Emotional intelligence organization

www.casel.org/Goleman.htm
A commercial site on emotional intelligence

www.21learn.org
The 21st Century Learning Initiative

www.aptt.com/
Edward De Bono training organization

www.snow.utoronto.ca/Learn2/sitemap.html
Good Learning to Learn site

Publishers and bookstores

www.brainstore.com
Bookseller specializing in brain-based learning

www.newhorizons.org/blab.html
Publisher selling material to do with brain-based learning

www.newhorizons.org
A publisher specializing in brain-based learning

www.scilearn.com
Scientific Learning Corporation

www.cainelearning.com/
Brain-based learning site with good links

Publications

http://archpsyc.ama-assn.org/
Archives of *General Psychiatry*

http://brain.oupjournals.org/
Oxford Journal of Neurology

www.beemnet.com/dana/
Dana Neuroscience Education resources

www.nature.com/neuro/
Nature neuroscience journal

www.sciencemag.org/
Science magazine

www.newscientist.com
New Scientist magazine

www.academicpress.com/nlm
Neurobiology of learning and memory

Ageing

www.alzheimers.org.uk/
Alzheimer's Disease Society

www.ama-assn.org/sci-pubs/journals
Archives of neurology gender differences in ageing

www.ageing.co.uk/
Research into ageing

Physiology and learning

www.bottledwater.org.
International Bottled Water Association

www.british-sleep-society.org.uk/
British Sleep Society

www.asdreams.org
International research group on dreams

www.braingym.org
Dennisons' Brain Gym® Organization

www.lboro.ac.uk/departments/hu/groups/sleep/
Sleep research laboratory, Loughborough

Learning difficulties

www.ldresources.com
Learning Disabilities Resources is a US online resource site

www.ldonline.org
Overview of learning disabilities

www.pavilion.co.uk/add/english.html
ADD links

www.add-adhd.org
ADD and ADHD

www.bda-dyslexia.org.uk/
British Dyslexia Association

www.interdys.org/
The International Dyslexia Association website

www.biausa.org/
Brain Injury Association

www.stroke.org.uk/
The Stroke Association

www.emmbrook.demon.co.uk/dysprax/homepage.htm
The Dyspraxia Foundation

Giftedness

www.nagcbritain.org.uk
National Association for Gifted Children

www.giftedl.uconn.edu/nrcgt.html
US National Research Centre for Gifted and Talented

www.cec.sped.org
US Council for Exceptional Children

www.edwebproject.org/edref.mi.intro.html
Multiple intelligences site

Gender difference in learning

www.science.ca/scientists/Kimura/kimura.html
Gender and brain organization

www.apa.org/releases/math2.html
Mathematics and gender

Research laboratories

inserm cnusc.fr:8113/cgi-bin
Stanislaus Dehaene's laboratory

www.boston-neurosurg.org
Neurosurgery – Brigham & Women's Hospital, Children's Hospital, Dana-
Farber Cancer Institute, Harvard Medical School

pzweb.harvard.edu/Research/Research
The official Harvard Project Zero site

uf3t.health.ufl.edu/csea/
Centre for the Study of Emotion and Attention

web-bcs.mit.edu/cgi-bin/faculty_page.pl?Name=spelke
Elizabeth Spelke's laboratory

www.psyc.bbk.ac.uk/cbcd/cbcd.html
Centre for the Brain and Cognitive Development, Birkbeck College

www.ion.ucl.ac.uk/
University College London Institute of Neurology

www.uci.edu/
University of California at Irvine

Institutes

www.ion.ucl.ac.uk/
Institute of Neurology

www.iop.kcl.ac.uk/IoP/index.stm
Institute of Psychiatry

www.mrc-cbu.cam.ac.uk/
Medical Research Council Cognition and Brain Sciences Unit

www.ninds.nih.gov/
National Institute of Neurological Disorders and Strokes

http://www.aan.com
American Academy of Neurology

www.bps.org.uk/
British Psychological Society

http://www.apa.org
American Psychological Association

http://www.winternet.com/~briminst
Institute for Brain and Immune Disorders

www.mrc.ac.uk/
Medical Research Council

Libraries and databases

www.brainland.com
Neuroscience information

www.washingtonopenmri.com/a2.htm
Open MRI brain scan

www.pnas.org/
Proceedings of the National Academy of Sciences

www.nih.gov/news/stemcell/primer.htm
Stem cell information

www.hhmi.org/senses/
Seeing, Hearing and Smelling the World

thalamus.wustl.edu/course/
Online neuroscience tutorial

www.med.harvard.edu/AANLIB/
The Whole Brain Atlas

www.vh.org/Providers/Textbooks/BrainAnatomy/BrainAnatomy.html
Virtual hospital brain anatomy

Music and learning

www.mozartcenter.com/index.html
Tomatis method

www.musica.uci.edu/
MuSICA Music & Science Information Computer Archive

www.mindinst.org/
MIND Institute Research into the Mozart Effect and Education

www.mri.ac.uk/index.html
UK-based music research centre

www.srpmme.u-net.com/
Society for Research in Psychology of Music and Music Education

Chapter 17

Glossary of terms

ACTH	A hormone that produces the long-term reaction to something stressful in the environment.
Adrenaline	A hormone that stimulates glucose release as a way of dealing with short-term stress. Also known as epinephrine.
Agnosia	Literally 'not knowing', agnosia is the condition of not recognizing sensory stimuli. For example, someone with visual agnosia would have no trouble seeing an object, but lacks the ability to understand the image.
Alzheimer's Disease	A degenerative, age-related form of dementia.
Amnesia	A cognitive disorder involving memory loss, typically as a result of a traumatic injury or a degenerative brain condition.
Amygdala	A part of the basal ganglia named for its almond shape. The amygdala is thought to be involved with emotion and memory formation.
Androgens	The 'male' hormones produced in the testes, including testosterone.
Angular Gyrus	A section of the left temporal lobe involved in language processing; it connects the occipital cortex with Wernicke's area.
Anterior	Front
Anterior Cingulate Gyrus	An area of the brain associated with motor control, pain perception, cognitive function and emotional arousal. A component of the limbic system.
Aphasia	Partial or total loss of the ability to express ideas or comprehend spoken or written language, resulting from damage to the brain caused by injury or disease.
Attention	The selection of stimuli to which we direct conscious thought.
Attention-Deficit Hyperactivity Disorder (ADHD)	A syndrome characterized by short attention span and poor impulse control.
Auditory Feedback	The process by which humans learn to speak utilizing hearing and vocalization. In auditory feedback sounds heard are repeatedly mimicked and fine tuned until they can be perfectly reproduced.

Autonomic Nervous System	Also called the visceral nervous system. Located outside the brain and spinal cord. Obtains sensory information from internal organs and provides output to them.
Axon	An extension of a neural cell that transports information to and from the cell body, usually by an electrical impulse.
Basal Ganglia	A series of subcortical structures in the centre of the brain that are principally responsible for motor tasks.
Blind Spot	A spot in the visual field of each eye where the eye cannot see. The blind spot corresponds to the point in the retina where the optic nerve exits the eye and which is devoid of photoreceptors.
Brain Stem	The major route by which the forebrain communicates with the spinal cord and peripheral nerves. The brain stem controls, among other things, respiration and regulation of heart rhythms.
Broca's Area	The central region for the production of speech. Located in the frontal lobe, typically in the left hemisphere.
Central Executive	A component of the working memory models associated with co-ordinating cognitive functions.
Chromosome	Thread-like structure of the cell nucleus that contains genetic information; they occur in characteristic matched pairs for each species humans have 23 pairs.
Central Nervous System (CNS)	The 'Central Station' to which the peripheral and visceral (autonomic) systems send their sensory information. The CNS takes that sensory information and responds to the peripheral and visceral systems with motor instructions. The two main structures of the CNS are the brain and the spinal cord.
Cerebellum	A large structure located high inside the hindbrain. Connected to the pons, medulla, spinal cord and thalamus. Helps control movement and some aspects of motor learning.
Cerebral Cortex	The outer, highly convoluted layer of the cerebral hemispheres. Responsible for perception, emotion, thought and planning.
Cerebral Hemispheres	The halves of the brain, each with its own specific functions. The left hemisphere is typically associated with speech, writing, language and calculation, and the right hemisphere is typically associated with spatial perception, visual recognition, and aspects of music perception and production.
Cerebral Palsy	A developmental disorder characterized by motor control difficulties; cerebral palsy results from perinatal damage to brain tissue.

Cingulate Gyrus	A cortical structure, part of the limbic system, that is directly over the corpus callosum along the medial side of each hemisphere. It is involved with regulating emotion and attention and in 'tagging'.
Circadian Rhythms	The basic rest–activity cycle. Regulated by a structure in the brain known as the suprachiasmatic nucleus (SCN) that determines levels of wakefulness over a 24-hour period.
Cognition	The mental processes by which knowledge or awareness is applied to comprehension and problem solving.
Cognitive Interference	The theory that certain cognitive processes in the brain may conflict with other cognitive processes.
Cognitive Map Theory	One theory concerning how the brain represents physical spaces.
Consciousness	One's immediate awareness. Consciousness is arguably what makes us human. A highly controversial field of study, it is also an area where no one theory prevails. Being able to understand, self-regulate and share one's own thoughts are at the core of consciousness.
Contralateral	Related to the opposite side, as when functions on the right side of the body are controlled by the left side of the brain.
Corpus Callosum	A large bundle of nerve fibres that connects the left and right cerebral hemispheres.
Cortical Plasticity	The ability for connections between neurons to be modified within the cortex.
Corticospinal Tract	Direct pathway from the cortex to the spine, involved in voluntary motor control.
Cortisol	A long-term stress hormone that maintains blood pressure and produces glucose for energy at times of stress.
Decussation	A crossing over of nerve fibre tracts from one side of the body's midline to the other. Typically result in the right hemisphere of the brain controlling the left side of the body, and the left hemisphere controlling the right side of the body.
Dendrite	A branching extension from the neuron cell body that receives information from other neurons.
Deoxyribonucleic Acid (DNA)	A long, thread-like molecule contained in the nucleus of cells that encodes the genetic information of an organism. DNA is a remarkable molecule because it can self-replicate. Half of a child's DNA contains genetic information from the mother and half from the father.

Dopamine	A neuromodulator acting principally through structures of the basal ganglia. Dopamine is associated with reward pathways, and low levels of dopamine are characteristic of Parkinson's disease.
Dorsal	In humans, closer to the back of the body.
Dorsolateral Pre-frontal Cortex	An area on the lateral aspect of the brain near the front that is associated with executive function, decision making and working.
Dyscalculia	A disability in mathematical calculation.
Dyslexia	A disability that inhibits reading and writing.
Dyspraxia	A disability in voluntary movement that also impacts on general learning abilities.
Epilepsy	A neurological disorder caused by uncontrolled electrical activity that spreads throughout the brain, causing seizures that can last from seconds to several minutes.
Episodic Memory	A type of long-term memory that references events and time.
Executive Processes	Cognitive tasks related to decision making, associated with the frontal lobe of the brain.
Frontal Cortex	An area of the brain associated with higher cognitive functions including planning and motor control.
Frontal Lobe	One of the four divisions of each hemisphere of the cerebral cortex that include the parietal, temporal and occipital. The site of emotions, personality, cognitive and motor functions.
Functional Magnetic Resonance Imaging (fMRI)	A technique for imaging brain activity using magnets.
Gene	The smallest hereditary unit. A gene is a section of DNA that encodes a protein and proteins in turn control many characteristics of an organism.
Glial Cells	A range of cell types that act to support the neural network by providing structure and nourishment. In some cases, glia may be involved in modulating neural signals.
Glucocorticoids	Any of a group of steroid hormones that affect glucose metabolism.
Hemisphere	Half of the brain, the right or left.
Hippocampus	A cortical structure near the centre of the brain that plays an important role in memory. The hippocampus is named for its seahorse-like shape in cross-section.

Hypothalamus	The master control structure for the autonomic nervous system and the secretion of hormones.
Inferior Colliculus	A cluster of cells responsive to sound. Found in the brain stem below the superior colliculus.
Inhibitory	Referring to a synaptic connection that decreases the electrical excitability of the postsynaptic neuron.
Ipsilateral	Opposite side, for example, right hemisphere controlling movement on the left side of the body.
Kinaesthesia	The sense by which muscular motion, weight, position, etc., are perceived.
Lateral	Referring to a structure that is closer to the side or surface of another structure, as opposed to medial. For example, the lateral part of an egg is the egg white, and the medial part is the yolk.
Limbic System	A group of brain structures that work to regulate emotions, memory and certain aspects of movement. Includes the amygdala, hippocampus, cingulate gyrus, septum and basal ganglia.
Long-Term Potentiation (LTP)	A long-lasting increase in the efficacy of a synapse.
Longitudinal Fissure	A deep sulcus (groove) that runs down the middle of the cortex and provides a prominent landmark for separating the brain into the left and right hemispheres.
Magnetic Resonance Imaging (MRI)	A technique for imaging soft tissues, especially the brain, using magnets. While MRI provides a static image of the brain, a related technique called fMRI (functional magnetic resonance imaging) can image changing activity within the brain.
Medial	Referring to a structure that is closer to the midline of another structure, as opposed to a lateral. For example, the medial part of an egg is the yolk, while the lateral part is the egg white.
Medulla Oblongata (Myelencephalon)	Located within the brain stem, or hindbrain. Responsible for controlling respiration, circulation and other bodily functions.
Melatonin	Hormone secreted by the pineal gland during the hours of darkness and which induces sleep.
Memory Space Theory	A theory of hippocampal function suggesting that the hippocampus acts to encode environmental episodes rather than spaces in particular. As opposed to the cognitive map theory.
Modality	A mode of sensation, for example, hearing, touch, smell, taste or vision.

Myelin	A glassy, white sheath surrounding the axons of some neurons. Myelin acts as an insulator, and helps neural signals travel more quickly and over greater distances than they could in an uninsulated axon. Myelin is composed of Schwann cells that wrap themselves concentrically around the neural axon.
Neglect	The slow demise of a system.
Neo-cortex	Literally meaning 'new cortex,' because it evolved later than other brain areas. Located in the dorsal, or front part of the brain, the neocortex is especially large in higher primates and is responsible for sensory and motor processing as well as abstract reasoning and association.
Neonate	Newly born.
Neuron	The cellular unit of the central and peripheral nervous systems.
Neurotransmitter	A chemical released by neurons to relay information to other cells.
Noradrenaline	A short-term stress hormone that works in conjunction with adrenaline. It also impairs short-term memory and scientists now believe it can promote the growth of bacteria. It also gives you a short-lived feeling of alertness.
Nucleus Acccumbens	Principal pleasure centre in the brain, containing one of the highest stores of dopamine. Highly involved in motivation and reward systems. Studied extensively by those involved in addiction research.
Occipital Lobe	Located at the back of the brain. Mostly devoted to vision. Contains the primary visual cortex.
Oestrogen	High levels of this hormone are present in women and lower levels in men. It helps define 'femaleness' and is involved in creating female body shape.
Olfactory	Of or relating to the sense of smell.
Orbitofrontal Cortex (aka Brodmann's Area 47)	A region of the frontal cortex that is involved in motor function and communicates with the basal ganglia as well as other limbic structures. This structure may be involved in mood-related disorders as well as motor dysfunction.
Parietal Lobe	Contains somatosensory areas and sensory integration areas. Separated from the frontal lobe by the central sulcus, and from the occipital lobe by the parieto-occipital sulcus.
Pathway	A route of information flow in the nervous system.
Perinatal	Relating to the time just before, during, and just after birth.

Peripheral Nervous System	Located outside the brain and spinal cord. Obtains sensory information from the external world and provides motor output to the voluntary muscles that allow us to move.
Phonemes	The smallest recognizable speech sounds and root of all spoken language. When added together, phonemes create syllables, which allows the creation of words.
Pituitary Gland	A small gland at the base of the brain that secretes hormones that regulate most of the other glands in the body. Often referred to as the 'master gland'.
Planum Temporale	A cluster of neurons believed to be important for language processing; in most people, it is larger in the left hemisphere than in the right.
Pons	A structure at the top of the brain stem containing a number of nuclei and many fibre tracts connecting the cerebellum and medulla to the higher brain areas.
Posterior	Rear
Posterior Parietal Cortex	Posterior portion of the parietal cortex involved in transforming visual information to motor commands.
Positron Emission Tomography (PET)	A technique for imaging brain activity using radioactive dyes injected into the bloodstream.
Postsynaptic	On the receiving side of the synapse. A postsynaptic cell receives neurotransmitter from a presynaptic neuron.
Pre-Frontal Cortex	An area of the brain associated with higher cognitive functions including planning and working memory.
Pre-Motor Cortex	Region of cortex in the frontal lobe involved in the sensory guidance of movement and activating proximal and trunk muscles.
Prenatal	Relating to the time before birth.
Primary Motor Cortex	Cortical area in the frontal lobe that is directly involved in producing muscle contraction.
Primary Visual Cortex	Located in the occipital lobe. Receives the earliest information from the eyes by way of the thalamus.
Procedural Memory	A type of unconscious memory for motor skills that does not require the hippocampus for formation.
Prosopagnosia	An inability to recognize faces following brain injury.
Psychometric	Measurement of mental processes.
REM Sleep	Rapid eye movement sleep. A phase of sleep in which it is thought some consolidation of memory and therefore learning occurs.

Saccadic Eye Movements	High velocity eye movements from one point to another point. When primates pan their gaze over a scene, their eyes move in saccades rather than in a continuous, smooth motion.
Serotonin	The oldest neurotransmitter in the brain; important for emotional processing and sleep.
Slow-Wave Sleep	A phase of sleep that is particularly deep.
Somatic Nervous System	Also called the voluntary nervous system, the somatic nervous system is a component of the peripheral nervous system that controls voluntary actions by carrying signals to skeletal muscles to make them contract.
Somatosensory	Relating to information perceived through sensory organs in the skin and muscles including tactile, temperature, pressure and position information.
Stress	Physical, emotional or mental pressure. In the context of this book, anything from the outside world that tips us out of homeostatic balance.
Stroke	A sudden, acute attack or injury.
Stroop Task	A test that measures cognitive interference, the role that one stimulus characteristic plays in the perception of another characteristic. The Stroop Effect is an increase in reaction time evident when a subject has to identify one stimulus property that conflicts with a more salient stimulus property. For example, if the word 'blue' is written in red ink, a subject will have a hard time identifying the ink colour.
Subcortical	Literally located beneath the cortex, referring to brain structures that are not a part of the cerebral cortex.
Supplementary Motor Area (SMA)	Region of cortex in the frontal lobe involved in the planning of complex movements and in two-handed movements.
Synapse	The physical structure that makes an electrochemical connection between two neurons.
Temporal lobe	Primarily responsible for hearing and memory/learning. Separated from the frontal lobe by the lateral sulcus.
Testosterone	The hormone that defines 'maleness'. It has been linked – controversially – with male aggressiveness, male libido and impatience. Males who are victims of violence suffer a significant drop in testosterone levels. Stress also lowers testosterone levels.
Thalamus	A structure in the brain that traffics sensory information such as vision, hearing and touch coming into the brain and distributes that information to appropriate areas of the cerebral cortex.

Visual Cortex	Any area of the cerebral cortex principally associated with vision.
Voluntary Nervous System	Also called the somatic nervous system, the voluntary nervous system is a component of the peripheral nervous system that controls voluntary actions by carrying signals to skeletal muscles to make them contract.
Wernicke's Area	An area of the left temporal lobe that is crucial for language comprehension.
Working Memory	A type of memory where information is readily available for a very short period of time.

Endnotes

1   Sylwester, Robert (2000) 'On teaching brains to think: a conversation with Robert Sylwester', Educational Leadership, ASCD, 57(7): 72

2   Bruer, John T. (1998) A Bridge Too Far

3   Carter, Rita (1999) Mapping the Mind, London , Weidenfeld and Nicolson

4   Gazzaniga, M. (1998) The Mind's Past, Berkeley, CA: University of California Press, quoted in Ratey, John (2001) A User's Guide to the Brain: Perception, Attention, and the Four Theaters of the Brain, Little Brown and Company, London, p. 288

5   Gazzaniga, M The Mind's Past quoted in Ratey, John (2001) A User's Guide to the Brain: Perception, Attention, and the Four Theaters of the Brain, Little Brown and Company, London, p.288

6   Thinking about the educational implications of genetics research will be a hugely important task for the future. The jump from gene to behaviour is much greater than the jump from brain to behaviour. The work to be done in terms of bringing neuroscience into contact with education will facilitate the work that will eventually have to be done to bring insights from genetics to bear on teaching and learning.

7   B. Devlin, Michael Daniels, Kathryn Roeder 'The heritability of IQ' Nature 388, 468–471 (31 Jul 1997)

8   Yale Bulletin and Calendar, 20 October 2000, 29(7). See http://www.yale.edu/opa/v29.n7/story4.html

9   Yale Bulletin and Calendar, 20 October 2000, 29(7). See http://www.yale.edu/opa/v29.n7/story4.html

10 Herzmann, C., Torrens J. K., de Escobar, G. M., et al. (1999) 'Maternal thyroid deficiency during pregnancy and subsequent neuropsychological development of the child', N Engl J Med, 23 December, 341: 2015–17

11 BUPA Health News Journal, 3 September 2001. See http://www.bupa.co.uk/health_news/030901pregnancy.html

12 Brain in the News, 15 November 1997, 4(11): 4

13 See http://www.icn.ucl.ac.uk/members/Csibr25/

14 Haber, R. N. and Levin, C. A. (1989) 'The lunacy of moon watching: some preconditions to an explanation of the moon illusion', in M. Hershenson (ed.) The Moon Illusion, Hinsdale, NJ: Lawrence Erlbaum Associates, 299–318

15 Müller, Matthias M., Herrmann, Christoph S., Friederici, Angela D., Csibra, G. and Johnson, M. H. (2001) 'Object processing in the infant brain', Science, 13 April, 292: 163

16 Professor Alison Gopnik, Brain Expo, San Diego, 4 January 2001

17   DeCasper, A. J. and Fifer, W. P. (1980) 'Of human bonding: newborns prefer their mother's voice', Science, 208: 1174-6

18   See Harris, P. (1989) Children and Emotion, Oxford: Blackwell

19   Field, T. M., Cohen, D., Garcia, R. and Greenberg, R. (1984). 'Mother-stranger face discrimination by the newborn', Infant Behaviour and Development, 7: 19-25

20   Rizzolatti, G., Gentilucci, M., Camarda, R. M., et al. (1990) 'Neurons relating to reaching-grasping arm movements in the rostral part of area 6 (area 6a beta)', Experimental Brain Research, 82: 337-50

21   See also Blakemore, S.-J. and Frith, U. (2000) The Implications of Recent Developments in Neuroscience for Research on Teaching and Learning, ESRC Teaching and Learning Research Programme for an argument in favour of modelling in learning

22   Harris, Judith Rich (1998) The Nurture Assumption: Why Children Turn out the Way They Do, London: Bloomsbury

23   Meltzoff, A. N. (1999) 'Persons and representation: why infant imitation is important for theories of human development', in J. Nadel and G. Butterworth (eds), Imitation in Infancy, Cambridge: Cambridge University Press, 9-35. See also Iacoboni, M., Woods, R. P., Brass, M., Bekkering, H., Mazziotta, J. C. and Rizzolatti, G. (1999) 'Cortical mechanisms of human imitation', Science, 286: 2526-8

24   Gopnik, A., Meltzoff, A. and Kuhl, P. (1999) How Babies Think, London: Weidenfeld and Nicolson. Also see Eliot, Lise (1999) What's Going On In There? How the Brain and Mind Develop in the First Five Years of Life, New York: Bantam Books

25   http://www.psy.jhu.edu/faculty/jusczyk.html

26   Author notes of talk given at The Royal Institution, 'The development of the brain and early years learning', 16 November 2000

27   See Kotulak, Ronald (1996) Inside the Brain: Revolutionary Discoveries of How the Mind Works, Kansas: Andrews and McMeel

28   Author notes from the Royal Institution Seminars 'What can Brain Science tell us about Learning?', led by Sir Christopher Ball 21 September 2000

29   Susan Greenfield, Professor of Pharmacology, Oxford University, author notes from a talk given to the Technology Colleges Trust at the Royal Society, May 2000

30   Gage, Fred, Brain in the News, 15 April 1997, 4(4): 1

31   Greenfield, Susan (1999) Brain Power: Working out the Human Mind, London: Element Books, 28-9

32   Huttenlocher, P.R. (1993) 'Morphometric Study of Human Cerebral Cortex Development' in Brain Development and Cognition; A Reader, Mark H Johnson ed, Cambridge MA: Blackwell

      also Huttenlocher, P.R. (1987) 'The development of Synapses in Striate Cortex of Man,' Human Neurobiology, 6 1-9

      also Huttenlocher, P.R. (1979) 'Synaptic Density in Human Frontal Cortex': Development Changes and Effects of Aging', Brain Research 163 195-205

33   Author notes from States of Jersey, Learning in the 21st Century Conference,
      13 September 2001, quoted by John Abbot from Quartz and Sejnowski , The Salk
      Institute, The Neural Basis of Cognitive Development: a Constructivist Manifesto

34   Author notes from interview at the McLean Medical School, Boston, August 1999

35   Psychiatric News, May 2000; Computer Graphics World, January 2000; The Dana
      Foundation Magazine, Brainwork, January 2000;
      http://www.loni.ucla.edu/~thompson/MEDIA/media.html

36   Everhart, D. Erik, Shucard, Janet L., Quatrin, Teresa and Shucard, David W. (2001)
      'Sex-related differences in event-related potentials, face recognition, and facial
      affect processing in prepubertal children', Neuropsychology, 15(3)

37   Thompson, P.M., et al. (2000) 'Growth patterns in the developing brain detected by
      using continuum mechanical tensor maps', Nature, 204: 190–3

38   Blakemore, Sarah-Jayne and Frith, Uta (2000) The Implications of Recent
      Developments in Neuroscience for Research on Teaching and Learning, Institute of
      Cognitive Neuroscience, 17 Queen Square, London WC1N 3BG. Email:
      s.blakemore@ucl.ac.uk and u.frith@ucl.ac.uk

39   Goleman, Daniel (1998) Emotional Intelligence: Why It Can Matter More Than IQ,
      London: Bloomsbury

40   Author notes from a talk entitled 'Memory, Brain, Self and Culture,' by Professor
      Martin Conway given at The Institute for Cultural Research, London University,
      Memory Matters Seminars, 16-17 February 2002

41   MacLean, Paul (1990) The Triune Brain in Evolution, Plenum Publishers

42   Simons, D. J. (2000) 'Current approaches to change blindness', Visual Cognition:
      Special Issue on Change Detection and Visual Memory, 7: 1–16. See
      http://www.wjh.harvard.edu/~dsimons/

43   Pert, Candace (1997) The Molecules of Emotion, New York: Touchstone Books,
      144–6

44   Sylwester, Robert (1999) 'In search of the roots of adolescent aggression',
      Educational Leadership, September: 65. Also from author notes from a presentation
      given to the Brain Expo 2000, San Diego, 16 January 2000.

      See also Le Doux, Joseph (1996) Emotional Brain, New York: Simon and Schuster

45   Ratey, John (2001) A User's Guide to the Brain: Perception, Attention, and the Four
      Theaters of the Brain, Little Brown and Company, London p223

46   Zohar, Danah and Marshall, Ian (2000) Spiritual Intelligence: The Ultimate
      Intelligence, London: Bloomsbury

47   Quoted Blakemore, S.-J. and Frith, U. (2000) The Implications of Recent
      Developments in Neuroscience for Research on Teaching and Learning, ESRC
      Teaching and Learning Research Programme. 'Other functional imaging studies have
      associated financial reward with activation of ventral striatum, midbrain, thalamic,
      and pre-frontal regions (Thut et al., 1997).'

48   Damasio (1994) Descarte's Error: Emotion, Reason and the Human Brain, New York,
      Putnam

49   Meyer, G., Hauffa, B. P.; Schedlowski, M., Pawlak, C., Stadler, M. A., Exton, M. S. (2000) 'Casino gambling increases heart rate and salivary cortisol in regular gamblers', Biological Psychiatry, 48(9), 948–53

50   Elliott, R., Friston, K. J. and Dolan, R. J. (2000) 'Dissociable neural responses in human reward systems', Journal of Neuroscience, 20(16): 6159–65

51   Le Doux, Joseph (1996) Emotional Brain, New York: Simon and Schuster

52   Damasio, Antonio (2000) The Feeling of What Happens: Body and Emotion in the Making of Consciousness, London: Vintage

53   See Sternberg, R. J. (1988) The Triarchic Mind: A New Theory of Human Intelligence, New York: Viking; Sternberg, R. J. (1996) Successful Intelligence: How Practical and Creative Intelligence Determine Success in Life, New York: Plume

54   Professor David Gold and Dr Ewan McNay, University of Virginia, published in Proceedings of the National Academy of Sciences and the journal Neurobiology of Learning and Memory.

55   Nichelli, P., Grafman, J., Pietrini, P., Alway, D., Carton, J. C. and Miletich, R. (1994) 'Brain activity during chess playing', Nature, 369(6477): 191

56   Educational Leadership, November 2001, 59(3) Wired For Mathematics: A Conversation with Brian Butterworth, Marcia D'Arcangelo, p14-19

57   Dehaene, S. (1997) The Number Sense: How the Mind Creates Mathematics, London: Allen Lane – Penguin Press; for Elizabeth Spelke see http://www.news.harvard.edu/gazette/2001/11.29/03-spelke.html

58   Dehaene, S., Dehaene-Lambertz, G. and Cohen, L. (1998) 'Abstract representations of numbers in the animal and human brain', Trends in Neuroscience, 21(8): 355-61. Also Dehaene, S., Spelke, E., Pinel, P., Stanescu, R. and Tsivkin, S. (1999) 'Sources of mathematical thinking: behavioral and brain-imaging evidence', Science, 284(5416): 970-4

59   London Observer, 19 August 2001, 7

60   Rauscher, Shaw and Ky (1993) 'Music and spatial task performance', Nature, 365/6447; see also Rauscher, Shaw and Ky (1995) 'Listening to Mozart enhances spatial temporal reasoning: toward a neurophysiological basis', Neuroscience Letters, 185: 4–7; also Rauscher, Shaw, Levine, Ky and Wright (1994) 'Music and spatial task performance: a causal relationship', paper to the American Psychological Association 102nd Annual Convention, Los Angeles

61   Weinberger and McKenna (1990) 'Sensitivity of single neurons in auditory cortex to contour', Music Perception, 5

62   Chan, Agnes S., Ho, Yim-Chi, and Cheung, Mei-Chun (1998) 'Music training improves verbal memory', Nature, 396: 128

63   Pantev, C., Oostenveld, R., Engelien, A., Ross, B., Roberts, L. E. and Hoke, M. (1998) 'Increased auditory cortical representation in musicians', Nature, 392: 811-4

64   Pascual-Leone, A., Nguyet, D., Cohen, L. G., Brasil-Neto, J. P., Cammarota, A. and Hallett, M. (1995) 'Modulation of muscle responses evoked by transcranial magnetic stimulation during the acquisition of new fine motor skills', Journal of Neurophysiology, 74(3): 1037–45

65   'What the brain tells us about music: amazing facts and astounding implications revealed', MRN, Fall 2000

66   See Hurwitz, I., Wolff, P. H., Bortnick, B. D. and Kokas, K. (1975) 'Nonmusical effects of the Kodaly music curriculum in primary grade children', Journal of Learning Disabilities, 8: 45–51; Frith, U. (1985) 'Beneath the surface of developmental dyslexia', in K. E. Patterson, J. C. Marshall and M. Coltheart (eds), Surface Dyslexia, Hove: Lawrence Erlbaum Associate Ltd, 301–30; Lamb, S. J. and Gregory, A. H. (1993) 'The relationship between music and reading in beginning readers', Educational Psychology, 13: 19–26

67   Kastner, Sabine, De Weerd, Peter, Desimone, Robert and Ungerleider, Leslie (1999) Science, 2 October

68   Jeannerod, M. (1994) 'The representing brain – neural correlates of motor intention and imagery', Behavioral and Brain Sciences, 17: 187–202

69   Yue, G. H., Bilodeau, M., Hardy, P. A., Enoka, R. M. (1997) 'Task-dependent effects of limb immobilization on the fatigability of the elbow flexor muscles in humans', Experimental Physiology, 82: 567–92; Yue, G. H., Ranganathan, V. K., Siemionow, V., Sahgal, V. (1999) 'Older adults exhibit a reduced ability to maximally activate their elbow flexor muscles', Journal of Gerontology: Medical Sciences, 54: M249–53; Yue, G. H., Liu, J. Z., Siemionow, V., Ranganathan, V. K., Sahgal, V. (in press) 'Brain activation during human finger extension and flexion movements', Brain Research; also see http://www.lerner.ccf.org/pi/gyue.html

70   Ratey, John (2001) A User's Guide to the Brain: Perception, Attention, and the Four Theaters of the Brain, London: Little Brown and Company, p. 189–90

71   Professor Kim Plunkett from author notes of talk at The Royal Institute, 'The development of the brain and early years learning', 16 November 2000

72   Scientists at Duke University publishing findings in Brain Research October 2000

73   Barkley, R. A. (1997) ADHD and the Nature of Self-control, New York: Guilford Press. Also Barkley, R. A. (1998) Attention-Deficit Hyperactivity Disorder: A Handbook for Diagnosis and Treatment, New York: Guilford Press

74   Ratey, John (2001) A User's Guide to the Brain: Perception, Attention, and the Four Theaters of the Brain, London: Little Brown and Company, p. 126

75   Barkley, R. A. (1998) Attention-Deficit Hyperactivity Disorder: A Handbook for Diagnosis and Treatment, New York: Guilford Press. Also http://www.sciam.com/1998/0998issue/0998barkley.html

76   Castellanos, F. Xavier, Giedd, Jay N., Berquin, Patrick C., et al. (2001) 'Quantitative brain magnetic resonance imaging in girls with Attention-Deficit/Hyperactivity Disorder', Archives of General Psychiatry, 58(3): March

77   Research done by Helene Gjone and Jon M. Sundet of the University of Oslo with Jim Stevenson of the University of Southampton with 526 identical twins, who inherit exactly the same genes, and 389 fraternal twins, who are no more alike genetically than siblings born years apart found that ADHD has a heritability approaching 80 per cent

78   Berk, Laura E.; 'Why Children Talk to Themselves,' by Scientific American, November 1994

79   Anderson, Steven W., Bechara, Antoine, Damasio, Hanna, Tranel, Daniel and Damasio, Antonio R. (1999) 'Impairment of social and moral behavior related to early damage in human prefrontal cortex', Nature Neuroscience, 2: 1032–7

80   See Kotulak, Ronald (1996) Inside the Brain: Revolutionary Discoveries of How the Mind Works, Kansas: Andrews and McMeel

81   Castro-Caldas, A., Petersson, K. M., Reis, A., Stone-Elander, S. and Ingvar, M. (1998) 'The illiterate brain. Learning to read and write during childhood influences the functional organization of the adult brain', Brain, 121(6): 1053–63; also from author notes from a talk given by Martin Ingvar at Birmingham NEC, 28 February 2002

82   Paulesu, E. and Mehler, J. (1998) 'Right on in sign language', Nature – News and Views, 392: 233–4

83   Torgesen, J. K., Alexander, A. W., Wagner, R. K., Rashotte, C. A., Voeller, K., Conway, T. and Rose, E. (2001) 'Intensive remedial instruction for children with severe reading disabilities: immediate and long-term outcomes from two instructional approaches' Journal of Learning Disabilities, 34: 33–58; Torgesen, J. K. and Mathes, P. (2000) A Basic Guide to Understanding, Assessing, and Teaching Phonological Awareness, Austin, TX: PRO-ED; Torgesen, J. K. (2000) 'Individual differences in response to early interventions in reading: the lingering problem of treatment resisters', Learning Disabilities Research and Practice, 15: 55–64; Torgesen, J. K. (1999) 'Phonologically based reading disabilities: toward a coherent theory of one kind of learning disability', in R. J. Sternberg and L. Spear-Swerling (eds), Perspectives on Learning Disabilities, New Haven: Westview Press, pp. 231–62

84   Author notes from conference 'Early Learning and the Brain' held at the Royal Institution London, 12 July 2000

85   Dr David Reynolds, Exeter University and on ITV Tonight, Trevor McDonald, 21 January 2002

86   Portwood, Madeleine (1999) Developmental Dyspraxia: Identification and Intervention, 2nd edn, London: David Fulton Publishing

87   Author notes from seminars 'Brain Research and Learning' held at the Royal Institution London, Spring 2000

88   'Stimulating environment protects brain cells', Nature Medicine, April 1999, 5: 448–53, (Reuters Health) Reuters

89   Author notes from conference 'Early Learning and the Brain' held at the Royal Institution London, 12 July 2000

90   Professor Robert Sapolsky, Stanford University, San Diego Conference, January 2000

91   http://www.researchmatters.harvard.edu/section_list.php?section=mind

92   'Cortisol levels during human ageing predict hippocampal atrophy and memory deficits', Nature Neuroscience, May 1998

93   Author notes from talk 'Stress, disease and memory', Brain Expo, San Diego, 17 January 2000

94   BBC News Online, Health, 9 November 1998. See http://news.bbc.co.uk/hi/english/health/newsid_211000/211032.stm

95 Bechara, A., Tranel, D., Damasio, H. and Damasio, A. R. (1996) 'Failure to respond autonomically to anticipated future outcomes following damage to the pre-frontal cortex', Cerebral Cortex, 6: 215–25. See also Bechara, A., Damasio, H., Damasio, A. R., Lee, G. P. (1999) 'Different contributions of the human amygdala and ventromedial pre-frontal cortex to decision-making', Journal of Neuroscience, 19(13): 5473–81

96 Coffey, C. Edward, Lucke, Joseph F., Saxton, Judith A., et al. (1998) 'Sex differences in brain ageing – a quantitative magnetic resonance imaging study', Archives of General Psychiatry, February, 55(2)

97 Nelson, M., Bakaliou, F. and Trivedi, A. (1994) 'Iron deficiency anaemia and physical and academic performance in adolescent girls from different ethnic backgrounds', British Journal of Nutrition, 72: 427–33; Ash, R. and Nelson, M. (1998) 'Iron status and cognitive function in UK adolescent girls', Proc Nutr Soc, 57: 81A; see also http://www.kcl.ac.uk/kis/schools/life_sciences/health/nutrition/mn.htm

98 BBC News Online 14 April 2000, see http://news.bbc.co.uk/hi/english/health/newsid_713000/713087.stm

99 Benton, D. (1997) 'Psychological effects of snacks and altered meal frequency - a comment', British Journal of Nutrition, 77: S118–20; Benton, D. and Parker, P. Y. (1998) 'Breakfast, blood glucose and cognition', American Journal of Clinical Nutrition, 67: 772S–778S; Benton, D., Slater, O. and Donohue, R. T. (in press) 'The influence of breakfast and a snack on memory and mood', Physiology and Behavior; see http://psy.swan.ac.uk

100 Maszuda, M., Liu, Y. et al. (1999) Diabetes, 48: 1801–6; see http://fmri.ufbi.ufl.edu/labnews.html

101 Quoted from a letter to the New Scientist, 20 October 2001, 2313: 109

102 BBC News Online, 25 January 2001, see http://news.bbc.co.uk/hi/english/health/newsid_1133000/1133308.stm

103 Cahill, L. and McGaugh, J. L. (1998) 'Mechanisms of emotional arousal and lasting declarative memory', Trends in Neurosciences, 21: 294–9; Hamann, S. B., Cahill, L. and Squire, L. R. (1997) 'Emotional perception and memory in amnesia', Neuropsychology, 11: 1–10

104 See Behavioural and Brain Sciences Special Issue on Sleep and Dreaming, Cambridge University Press, 2001 – http://cogsci.soton.ac.uk/harnad/bbs.html

105 Maquet, P., et al. (1996) 'Functional neuroanatomy of human rapid-eye-movement sleep and dreaming', Nature, 12 September, 383:163

106 Article 'Sleepless in Loughborough'. See http://www.lboro.ac.uk/departments/hu/groups/sleep/wellcome.htm

107 Author notes from talk 'How circadian rhythms and light impact the human brain', Brain Expo, San Diego, 19 January 2000

108 Hobson, J. Allan and Stickgold, Robert (1994) 'A Neurocognitive Approach to Dreaming', Consciousness and Cognition, 3(1):1–15; Stickgold, Robert, Pace-Schott, Edward and Hobson, J. Allan (1994) 'A new paradigm for dream research: mentation reports following spontaneous arousal from REM and NREM sleep recorded in a home setting', Consciousness and Cognition, 3(1):16–29. See http://home.earthlink.net/~sleeplab/stickgold.html

109 Born, Jan, Hansen, Kirsten, Marshall, Lisa, Mölle, Matthias and Fehm, Horst L. J. (1992) Clin Endocrinol Metab, 75: 1431–5; Mason, J. W., Hartley, L. H., Kotchen, T. A., Mougey, E. H., Ricketts, P. T. and Jones, L. G. (1973) 'Plasma cortisol and norepinephrine responses in anticipation of muscular exercise', Psychosom Med, 35: 406–14

110 J Dev and Behavioral Pediatrics (1999) 20: 28–33

111 Author notes from talk 'How circadian rhythms and light impact the human brain', Brain Expo, San Diego, 19 January 2000

112 Opie I and Opie P (1969) Games Children Play, OUP, London

113 Bekoff, Marrk (2001) 'Social play behaviour: co-operation, fairness, trust and the evolution of morality', Journal of Consciousness Studies, 8: 81. Also Iwaniuk, Nelson and Pellis (2001) 'Do big brained animals play more?', Journal of Comparative Psychology, 115: 29

114 Bryant Furlow, 'Play's the Thing', New Scientist 9 June 2001, 2294: 30

115 Op cit 28–31

116 Creativity Research Journal, 1999, 12: 129–39

117 Elbert, Thomas, Pantev, Christo, Wienbruch, Christian, et al. (1995) 'Increased cortical representation of the fingers of the left hand in string players', Science, 270: 305–7

118 Exeter Fit to Succeed Project, see http://www.sheu.org.uk/fts/ftspress.htm

119 See http://www.britassoc.org.uk; http://www.phoenix.herts.ac.uk/

120 See http://www.csulb.edu/~kmacd/laughter.htm

121 UCI Newsroom March 2001

122 Author notes from a talk given by Professor Robert Sapolsky, Stanford University, at the San Diego Conference, January 2000

123 See http://research.medicine.wustl.edu/ocfr/research.nsf.

124 Author notes from talk 'Stress, disease and memory', Brain Expo, San Diego, 17 January 2000. See also Sapolsky, Robert (1998) Why Zebras Don't Get Ulcers, New York: Freeman

125 Levine, S. (1971) 'Stress and behavior', Scientific American, 224(1): 26–31; Seligman, M., Rosellini, R. and Kozak, M. (1975) 'Learned helplessness in the rat', J Compar Physiol Psychol, 88: 542–7; Seligman, M. (1975) Helplessness, San Francisco: Freeman & Co

126 See http://www.nobel.se/medicine/laureates/1981/sperry-lecture.html, Nobel Lecture, 8 December 1981

127 Corballis, M.C. (1991) The Lopsided Ape: Evolution Of The Generative Mind, Oxford: OUP

128 Thatcher, R. W., Walker, R. A. and Guidice, S. (1987) 'Human cerebral hemispheres develop at different rates and ages', Science, 236: 1110–13

129 Guiard, Y. (1987) 'Asymmetric division of labor in human skilled bimanual action: The kinematic chain as a model', The Journal of Motor Behavior, 19(4): 486–517

130 Coren, S. and Halpern, D. F. (1991) 'Left-handedness: A marker for decreased survival fitness', Psychological Bulletin, 109: 99. See also http://duke.usask.ca/~elias/left/index.html for general information about left-handedness

131 Hannaford, Carla (1997) The Dominance Factor, Great Ocean Publishers

132 Benbow, C. P., Lubinski, D., Shea, D. L. and Eftekhari-Sanjani, H. (2000) 'Sex differences in mathematical reasoning ability: Their status 20 years later', Psychological Science, 11: 474–80; Benbow, C. P. (1990) 'Sex differences in mathematical reasoning ability: Further thoughts', Behavior and Brain Sciences, 13: 196; Benbow, C. P. and Arjmand, O. (1990) 'Predictors of high academic achievement in mathematics and science by mathematically talented students', Journal of Educational Psychology, 82: 430–41; Benbow, C. P. and Minor, L. L. (1990) 'Cognitive profiles of verbally and mathematically precocious students: Implications for identification of the gifted', Gifted Child Quarterly, 34: 21–6

133 Ornstein, Robert (1997) The Right Mind: Making Sense of the Hemispheres, London: Harcourt and Brace, 103

134 Brain in the News, 15 August 1997, 4(8): 5

135 Ramachandran, V. S, Blakeslee, S. and Sacks O. (1999) Phantoms in the Brain: Probing the Mysteries of the Human Mind, London: Fourth Estate

136 Brown, Hallie D. and Kosslyn, Stephen M. (1998) 'Hemispheric differences in visual object processing', in Davidson and Hugdahl (eds), Brain Asymmetry, Cambridge, MA: MIT Press, 93

137 Ratey, John (2001) A User's Guide to the Brain: Perception, Attention, and the Four Theaters of the Brain, Little Brown and Company, London p230

138 See Sapolsky, Robert (1998) Why Zebras Don't Get Ulcers, New York: Freeman

139 Cacioppo, John T., Tassinary, Louis G. and Berntson, Gary (eds) (2001) Handbook of Psychophysiology, 2nd edn, Cambridge: CUP

140 Quoted Springer, Sally P. and Deutsch, George (1998) Left Brain, Right Brain: Perspectives from Cognitive Neuroscience, New York: Freeman p104; Sasanuma, S., Itoh, M., Mori, K. and Kobayashi, Y. (1977) 'Tachistoscopic recognition of Kana and Kanji words', Neuropsychologia, 27: 547–53

141 Morton, L. L., Kershner, J. R. and Siegel, L. S. (1990) 'The potential for therapeutic applications of music on problems related to memory and attention', Journal of Music Therapy, 4(17): 195–208

142 Shuchard et al. (1990) 'Auditory evoked potentials and hand preference in 6 month old infants', Developmental Psychology, 26: 923–30

143 Hampson, 1990; 1995 quoted Blakemore, S.-J. and Frith, U. (2000) The Implications of Recent Developments in Neuroscience for Research on Teaching and Learning, ESRC Teaching and Learning Research Programme

144 Lewis, David Warren and Diamond Cleeves, Marian (1998) 'The influence of gonadal steroids on the asymmetry of the cerebral cortex', in Davidsonn and Hugdahl (eds), Brain Asymmetry, Cambridge, MA: MIT Press, 42

145 Quoted Springer, Sally P. and Deutsch, George (1998) Left Brain, Right Brain: Perspectives from Cognitive Neuroscience, New York: Freeman; 'Knowledge about individual and group differences in how people think, learn, and remember is essential for understanding human cognition and developing educational programmes and theories that can identify cognitive weakness and capitalize on cognitive strengths. The real enemy is the potential for misuse of knowledge, not the knowledge itself.'

Halpern, D. F. (1996) 'Changing data, changing minds: what the data on cognitive sex differences tell us and what we hear', Learning and Individual Differences, 8: 73–82

146 See http://www.mcmaster.ca/ua/opr/times/fall98/witelson.htm

147 Good, C. D., Johnsrude, I., Ashburner, J., Henson, R. N. A., Friston, K. and Frackowiak, R. S. J. (2000) 'Voxel-based morphometry analysis of 465 normal adult human brains', Neuroimage, 11(5): S607

148 Kimura, Doreen (1999) Sex and Cognition, Cambridge, MA: MIT, 32–3

149 Dr Joseph T. Lurito, Assistant Radiology Professor at Indiana University School of Medicine – from author notes of talk given at the Radiological Society of North America Annual Meeting 2001

150 Quoted Springer, Sally P. and Deutsch, George (1998) Left Brain, Right Brain: Perspectives from Cognitive Neuroscience, New York: Freeman p139

151 See Home Knowledge and Skills for Life – First result from PISA 2000 http://www.pisa.oecd.org/knowledge/home/intro.htm

152 Educational Leadership, November 2001, 59(3) Wired For Mathematics: A Conversation with Brian Butterworth, Marcia D'Arcangelo, p14–19

153 Discussions held with Professor John Williams in designing tests for the BBC Programme August 2001

154 Carr and Jessup, University of Georgia, 1997 quoted in BrainWork, 15 July 1997, 7(4): 6

155 Kimura, Doreen (1999) Sex and Cognition, Cambridge, MA: MIT, 37

156 Author notes from Opening Minds to Thinking Conference held at Keele University, 14 July 2000

157 Author notes from seminars on Brain Research and Learning held at the Royal Institution London, Spring 2000

158 Berns, G. S., Cohen, J. D. and Mintun, M. A. (1997) 'Brain regions responsive to novelty in the absence of awareness', Science, 276(5316): 1272–5

159 Baddeley, A. (1993) Your Memory: A Users Guide, London: Prion

160 Author notes from a talk entitled 'Eyewitness Testimony,' by Doctor Amina Memon given at The Institute for Cultural Research, London University, Memory Matters Seminars, 16-17 February, 2002

161 Professor Susan Greenfield commenting on the Exeter Fit for Life Project findings, Daily Telegraph

162 Ratey, John (2001) A User's Guide to the Brain: Perception, Attention, and the Four Theaters of the Brain, London: Little Brown and Company, p. 194

163 Damasio, Antonio (2000) The Feeling of What Happens: Body and Emotion in the Making of Consciousness, London: Vintage

164 Author notes from talk given to Technology Colleges Trust, Royal Institution, 1 February 2000

165 Cahill, L. (1996) 'The neurobiology of memory for emotional events: converging evidence from infra-human and human studies', in Function and Dysfunction in the Nervous System, Symposium 61, Vol. LXI, Cold Spring Harbor Press, 259-264

166 BrainWork, January/February 1997, 7(1): 9

167 Sacks, Oliver (1985) The Man Who Mistook His Wife for a Hat and Other Clinical Tales, New York: Simon & Schuster. See also http://www.oliversacks.com/home.shtml

168 Ratey, John (2001) A User's Guide to the Brain: Perception, Attention, and the Four Theaters of the Brain, Little Brown and Company, London, 185

169 Loftus, Elizabeth F. and Ketcham, Katherine (1994) The Myth of Repressed Memory, New York: St Martin's Press; Carry, Maryanne, Manning, Charles G., Loftus, Elizabeth F. and Sherman, Steven J. (1996) 'Imagination inflation: imagining a childhood event inflates confidence that it occurred', Psychonomic Bulletin and Review, 3(2): 208–14

170 Memon, A. and Wright, D. B. (2000) 'Factors influencing witness evidence', in J. McGuire, T. Mason and A. Ōkane (eds), Behaviour, Crime and Legal Processes: A Sourcebook, Chichester: John Wiley & Sons; Wright, D. B. and Davies, G. M. (1999) 'Eyewitness testimony', in F. T. Durso, R. S. Nickerson, R. W. Schvaneveldt, S. T. Dumais, D. S. Lindsay and M. T. H. Chi, (eds), Handbook of Applied Cognition, Chichester: John Wiley & Sons, 789–818; for eyewitness testimony see also http://www.psychology.iastate.edu/faculty/gwells/homepage.htm

171 See also Cahill, L. (1996) 'The neurobiology of memory for emotional events: converging evidence from infra-human and human studies', in Function and Dysfunction in the Nervous System, Symposium 61, Vol. LXI, Cold Spring Harbor Press, 259–64. Also http://darwin.bio.uci.edu/neurobio/Faculty/Cahill/cahill.htm

172 Author notes from a talk entitled 'Learn to Remember,' by Dominic O'Brien given at The Institute for Cultural Research, London University, Memory Matters Seminars, 16-17 February, 2002

173 Brain in the News, 15 January 1997, 4(1): 2

174 Maguire, E. A., Gadian, D. G., Johnsrude, I. S., et al. (2000). 'Navigation-related structural change in the hippocampi of taxi drivers', Proceedings of the National Academy of Science U.S., 97(8): 4398-403

175   Knut, K., Kampe, W., Frith, Chris D., Dolan, Raymond J. and Frith, Uta (2001)
      'Psychology: Reward value of attractiveness and gaze', Nature, 413: 589; Maguire,
      E. A., Frith, C. D. and Cipolotti, L. (2001) 'Distinct neural systems for the encoding
      and recognition of topography and faces', Neuroimage, 13(4): 743–50. See also
      http://www.icn.ucl.ac.uk/members/Kampe364/

176   Haber, R. N. (1998) 'Retrieving lost memories: a review of Erdelyi's Recovery of
      Unconscious Memories', Journal of Hypnosis, 32: 56–8; Haber, R. N. (1985) 'One
      hundred years of visual perception: an ahistorical perspective', in S. Koch and D. E.
      Leary (eds), A Century of Psychology as Science: Retrospectives and Assessments,
      New York: McGraw-Hill, 250–81; Haber, R. N. (1982) 'It's silly to equate imagery
      with learning', Journal of Mental Imagery, 6(1): 32–4; Haber, R. N. (1981) 'The
      power of visual perceiving', Journal of Mental Imagery, 5: 1–16. Reprinted in
      Journal of Visual/Verbal Languaging, 1983, 3: 9–19

177   See Blakemore, S.-J. and Frith, U. (2000) The Implications of Recent Developments
      in Neuroscience for Research on Teaching and Learning, ESRC Teaching and
      Learning Research Programme, available online at www.ex.ac.uk/esrc-tlrp. 'A
      common suggestion (Jonides et al., 1996) is that the areas activated during
      maintenance of verbal material, (left premotor cortex, supplementary motor cortex
      and right cerebellum, left inferior frontal cortex), comprise a network involved in
      speech production. This is consistent with the proposal that rehearsal of rote
      learned stimuli uses articulatory codes (Baddeley, 1986).'

Selected bibliography
by section

2 Pre-wiring: what happens to the brain in the womb

Diamond, M. (1988) *Enriching Heredity: The Impact of Environment on the Anatomy of the Brain*, New York: Free Press

Eliot, Lise (1999) *What's Going On In There? How the Brain and Mind Develop in the First Five Years of Life*, New York: Bantam Books

3 Wired to fire: brain development in the first five years

Blakemore, Sarah Jane (2000) 'Early Years Learning: a Report to the Parliamentary Office of Science and Technology', London, June

Gopnik, A., Meltzoff, A. and Kuhl, P. (1999) *How Babies Think*, London: Weidenfeld and Nicolson

Siegel, D.J. (1999) *The Developing Mind: Toward a Neurobiology of Interpersonal Experience*, New York: Guilford Press

4 Wired for desire: the brain and the onset of puberty

Dawkins, R. (1989) *The Selfish Gene*, Oxford: OUP

Harris, Judith Rich (1998) *The Nurture Assumption: Why Children Turn out the Way They Do*, London: Bloomsbury

Howard, Pierce J. (1994) *The Owner's Manual for the Brain – Everyday Applications from Mind-Brain Research*, Texas: Bard Press

Kotulak, Ronald (1996) *Inside the Brain*, Kansas: Andrews and McMeel

McCrone, John (1996) *Going Inside*, London: Faber and Faber

Ratey, John (2001) *A User's Guide to the Brain: Perception, Attention, and the Four Theaters of the Brain*, London: Little Brown and Company

Restak, Ronald (1980) *The Brain: The Last Frontier*, New York: Warner

Scientific American Book of the Brain – with an introduction by Antonio Damasio (1999) New York: Scientific American

5 Wired to inspire: the completion of brain development

Butterworth, Brian (2000) *The Mathematical Brain*, London: Papermac

Calvin, N. (1996) *How Brains Think: Evolving Intelligence Then and Now*, London: Weidenfeld and Nicolson

Carter, R. (1998) *Mapping the Mind*, London: Weidenfeld and Nicolson

Dehaene, S. (1997) *How the Mind Creates Mathematics*, London: Penguin

Greenfield, Susan (2000) *Brain Story*, London: BBC Publications

Greenfield, Susan (1997) *The Human Brain: A Guided Tour*, Science Masters

Hogarth, R. (2001) *Educating Intuition*, Chicago: University of Chicago Press

Perkins, David (1992) *Smart Schools*, New York: Free Press

Sacks, Oliver (1985) *The Man Who Mistook His Wife for a Hat and Other Clinical Tales*, New York: Simon & Schuster

Sternberg, Robert J. (ed.) (1997) *The Nature of Creativity*, Cambridge: Cambridge University Press

Zohar, Danah and Marshall, Ian (2000) *Spiritual Intelligence: The Ultimate Intelligence*, London: Bloomsbury

6 Wired to misfire: learning from dysfunction
Barkley, R.A. (1995) *Taking Charge of ADHD: The Complete Authoritative Guide for Parents*, New York: Guilford Press
Niehoff, D. (1999) *The Biology of Violence: How Understanding the Brain, Behaviour, and Environment Can Break the Vicious Circle of Aggression*, New York: Free Press
Volavka, J. (1995) *Neurobiology of Violence*, Washington: American Psychiatric Press
Walker, H. and Sylwester, R. (1991) 'Where is school along the path to prison?', *Educational Leadership*, ASCD, 49, September 14–17
Weiss, G. and Trokenberg Hechtman, L. (1993) *Hyperactive Children Grown Up*, New York: Guilford Press

7 Wired to retire: ageing and the brain
Heston, L. and White, J.A. (1991) *The Vanishing Mind*, New York: W.H. Freeman
Khalsa, D.S. (1997) *Brain Longevity*, London: Century
Vernon, M. (1992) *Reversing Memory Loss*, Boston: Houghton Mifflin Company

8 Physiology: how do we maintain the brain?
Carlson, N.R. (1991) *Physiology of Behaviour*, Boston: Allyn and Bacon
Druckman, D. and Bjork, R.A. (1991) *In the Mind's Eye: Enhancing Human Performance*. Washington: National Academy Press
Ha Ha: The Science of Laughter
Logue, A.W. (1991) *The Psychology of Eating and Drinking*. New York: W.H. Freeman
Portwood, Madeleine (1999) *Developmental Dyspraxia: Identification and Intervention*, 2nd edn, London: David Fulton Publishing
Shapiro, Francine (1995) *Eye Movement Desensitisation and Reprocessing*, New York: Guilford

9 Engagement: how do we arouse and direct the brain?
Csikszentmihalyi, M. (1990) *Flow: The Psychology of Optimal Experience*, New York: Harper Collins
Damasio, Antonio (2000) *The Feeling of What Happens: Body and Emotion in the Making of Consciousness*, London: Vintage
Goleman, Daniel (1996) *Emotional Intelligence: Why it Can Matter More than IQ*, London: Bloomsbury
Kalin, N.H. (1993) 'The neurobiology of fear', *Scientific American*, May, 195–205
Lewis, M. and Haviland-Jones J.M. (2000) *The Handbook of Emotions*, New York: Guilford Press
Le Doux, Joseph (1996) *Emotional Brain*, New York: Simon and Schuster
Parasraman, Raja (1999) *The Attentive Brain*, Boston: MIT Press
Pert, Candace (1997) *Molecules of Emotion*, New York: Scribner
Ramachandran, V.S, Blakeslee, S. and Sacks, O. (1999) *Phantoms in the Brain: Probing the Mysteries of the Human Mind*, London: Fourth Estate
Sapolsky, R. (1998) *Why Zebras don't get Ulcers: An Updated Guide to Stress, Stress Related Diseases, and Coping*, New York: Freeman
Van der Kolk, Bessel A. (1996) *Traumatic Stress: The Effects of Overwhelming Experience on Mind, Body and Society*, New York: Guilford Press

10 Laterality: how do we develop left and right?

Davidson, Richard J. and Hugdahl, Kenneth (1996) *Brain Asymmetry*, Boston: MIT Press

Hellige, Joseph B. (1993) *Hemispheric Asymmetry: What's Right and What's Left*, Cambridge, MA: Harvard University Press

Ornstein, Robert (1997) T*he Right Mind: Making Sense of the Hemispheres*, New York: Harcourt Brace

Springer, Sally P. and Deutsch, George (1998) *Left Brain, Right Brain: Perspectives from Cognitive Neuroscience*, New York: Freeman

11 Gender: how do we respect difference?

Kimura, Doreen (1999) *Sex and Cognition*, Boston: MIT Press

Moir, A. and Jessell, D. (1991) *Brain Sex: The Real Difference Between Men and Women*, New York: Carol

Rogers, Lesley (1999) *Sexing the Brain*, London: Weidenfeld and Nicolson

12 Memory: how do we remember?

Baddeley, A.D. (1986) *Working Memory*, Oxford: Oxford University Press

Gordon, Barry (1995) *Memory: Remembering and Forgetting in Everyday Life*, New York: Mastermedia

Hobson, J. (1988) *The Dreaming Brain*, New York: Basic Books

Luria, Alexander (1986) *The Mind of a Mnemonist: A Little Book about a Vast Memory*, Cambridge, MA: Harvard University Press

Mirsky, N. (1994) *The Unforgettable Memory Book*, London: BBC

Rubin, David C. (ed.) (1996) *Remembering Our Past: Studies in Autobiographical Memory*, Cambridge: Cambridge University Press

Rupp, Rebecca (1998) *Committed to Memory: How We Remember and Why We Forget*, London: Aurum Press

Schachter, Daniel (1996) *Searching For Memory: The Brain, The Mind, and The Past*, New York: Basic Books

Schachter, Daniel (2001) *The Seven Sins of Memory*, Boston: Houghton Mifflin

Further reading

Blackmore, S. (1999) *The Meme Machine*, Oxford: OUP

Blakemore, S.-J. (2000) *Early Years Learning*, Parliamentary Office of Science and Technology (POST) Report, available online at www.parliament.uk/post/pn140.pdf

Blakemore, S.-J. and Frith, U. (2000) *The Implications of Recent Developments in Neuroscience for Research on Teaching and Learning*, ESRC Teaching and Learning Research Programme, available online at www.ex.ac.uk/esrc-tlrp

Bloom, F.E. and Lazerson, A. (1988) *Brain, Mind and Behaviour*, New York: W.H. Freeman and Co

Brandt, Ron (2000) 'On teaching brains to think: a conversation with Robert Sylwester', *Educational Leadership*, ASCD, 57, 7, April

Brothers, L. (1997) *Friday's Footprint: How Society Shapes the Human Mind*, New York: OUP

De Bono, E. (1986) *CORT Thinking Programme*, Oxford: Pergamon

Elbert, Thomas, Pantev, Christo, Wienbruch, Christian et al. (1995) 'Increased cortical representation of the fingers of the left hand in string players', *Science*, 270, 305–307

Feuerstein, R., Rand, Y., Hoffman, M. and Miller, R. (1980) *Instrumental Enrichment*, Baltimore: University Park Press

Feuerstein, Reuven (1990) *Instrumental Enrichment*, Baltimore: University Park Press

de Fockert, J.W., Rees, G., Frith, C.D. Lavie, N. (2001) 'The role of working memory in visual selective attention', (abstract & PDF), *Science*, 2 March, 291, 1803–1806

Gardner, Howard (1993) *Frames of Mind: The Theory of Multiple Intelligences*, London: Fontana

Gardner, Howard (1993) *The Unschooled Mind*, London: Fontana

Gazzaniga, Michael (1992) *Nature's Mind*, New York: Penguin Books

Gazzaniga, Michael (1998) *The Mind's Past*, Berkeley, CA: University of California Press

Greenfield, Susan (2002) *Brain Story*, London: BBC

Kandel, E.R., Schwartz, J.H., Jessell, T.M. et al. (1995) *Essentials of Neural Science and Behaviour*, New York: Appleton and Lange

Maguire, E.A., Henson, R.N., Mummery, C.J. and Frith, C.D. (2001) 'Activity in prefrontal cortex, not hippocampus, varies parametrically with the increasing remoteness of memories', (abstract), *Neuroreport*, 5 March, 12(3), 441–444

Perkins, David (1995) *Outsmarting IQ: The Emerging Science of Learnable Intelligence*, New York: The Free Press

Pickup, G.J. and Frith, C.D. (2001) 'Theory of mind impairments in schizophrenia: symptomatology, severity and specificity', (abstract), *Psychol Med*, February, 31(2), 207–220

Posner, M.I. and Raichle, M.E. (1997) *Images of Mind*, New York: Scientific American Library

Sternberg, R.J. (1988) *The Triarchic Mind: A New Theory of Human Intelligence*, New York: Viking

Sternberg, R.J. (1996) *Successful Intelligence: How Practical and Creative Intelligence Determine Success in Life*, New York: Plume

Sylwester, Robert (1995) *A Celebration of Neurons: An Educator's Guide to the Human Brain*, Virginia: ASCD

Index

The suffix g denotes a definition in the Glossary.